A Book on Self Acceptance

CRAFTED BY SKRIUWER

Copyright © 2024 by Skriuwer.

All rights reserved. No part of this book may be used or reproduced in any form whatsoever without written permission except in the case of brief quotations in critical articles or reviews.

For more information, contact : **kontakt@skriuwer.com** (www.skriuwer.com)

TABLE OF CONTENTS

CHAPTER 1: UNDERSTANDING SELF-ACCEPTANCE

- *Defining genuine self-acceptance*
- *Seeing why acceptance matters for peace*
- *Beginning the journey with honest self-reflection*

CHAPTER 2: THE ROOTS OF LOW SELF-WORTH

- *Uncovering hidden beliefs about worth*
- *Examining how upbringing and culture affect self-image*
- *Starting the process of breaking old patterns*

CHAPTER 3: FACING NEGATIVE SELF-TALK

- *Spotting the inner critic and its triggers*
- *Replacing harsh thoughts with supportive ones*
- *Learning to respond kindly when self-doubt appears*

CHAPTER 4: EMBRACING OUR FLAWS

- *Accepting imperfection without guilt or shame*
- *Shifting from hiding flaws to seeing them as growth areas*
- *Using self-compassion to handle personal shortcomings*

CHAPTER 5: BUILDING A POSITIVE INNER VOICE

- *Encouraging self-talk vs. destructive criticism*
- *Practicing affirmations for daily confidence*
- *Developing a kinder mental environment*

CHAPTER 6: OVERCOMING SELF-DOUBT AND FEAR

- *Identifying common sources of insecurity*
- *Facing fears step by step*
- *Transforming doubt into determination*

CHAPTER 7: SETTING HEALTHY BOUNDARIES

- *Recognizing personal limits and needs*
- *Communicating boundaries with respect and clarity*
- *Protecting emotional well-being in close relationships*

CHAPTER 8: LEARNING SELF-COMPASSION

- *Being gentle with yourself during hard times*
- *Replacing shame with understanding and empathy*
- *Healing old wounds through self-forgiveness*

CHAPTER 9: LETTING GO OF PERFECTIONISM

- *Noticing when perfectionism disrupts growth*
- *Adopting a mindset that sees mistakes as lessons*
- *Finding freedom in "good enough" progress*

CHAPTER 10: HEALING FROM PAST HURT

- *Acknowledging emotional scars and their impact*
- *Using self-awareness to process painful memories*
- *Moving forward with renewed strength and hope*

CHAPTER 11: STRENGTHENING SELF-BELIEF

- *Building trust in your own abilities*
- *Celebrating evidence of past successes*
- *Overcoming criticism and self-sabotage*

CHAPTER 12: PRACTICING MINDFULNESS FOR INNER PEACE

- *Staying present instead of reliving worries*
- *Using breathing and body awareness to reduce stress*
- *Connecting mindfulness to daily self-acceptance*

CHAPTER 13: FINDING YOUR UNIQUE STRENGTHS

- *Recognizing everyday talents and traits*
- *Turning natural abilities into confidence boosters*
- *Using strengths to guide personal and career choices*

CHAPTER 14: DEALING WITH STRESS AND ANXIETY

- *Identifying triggers that spark worry or tension*
- *Balancing responsibilities with coping tools*
- *Seeking healthy outlets for built-up emotions*

CHAPTER 15: BUILDING SUPPORTIVE RELATIONSHIPS

- *Finding friends and partners who encourage growth*
- *Communicating needs and setting boundaries together*
- *Resolving conflicts in ways that deepen connections*

CHAPTER 16: DEVELOPING EMOTIONAL RESILIENCE

- *Bouncing back from difficulties instead of feeling stuck*
- *Learning to adapt when life changes unexpectedly*
- *Tapping into inner strength and outside support*

CHAPTER 17: MAINTAINING A GROWTH MINDSET

- *Viewing challenges as opportunities to learn*
- *Shifting from fixed expectations to ongoing progress*
- *Staying curious and open to new experiences*

CHAPTER 18: BALANCING SELF-CARE & RESPONSIBILITY

- *Protecting mental health while handling life's demands*
- *Creating sustainable routines for well-being*
- *Avoiding burnout through healthy boundary-setting*

CHAPTER 19: CARRYING SELF-ACCEPTANCE FORWARD

- *Integrating lessons learned into everyday habits*
- *Adapting self-acceptance strategies as life evolves*
- *Moving ahead with confidence and inner peace*

CHAPTER 1: UNDERSTANDING SELF-ACCEPTANCE

Self-acceptance is about recognizing who we are, appreciating our unique qualities, and making peace with our flaws. It involves an honest look at ourselves—our strengths, weaknesses, and everything in between. When we truly accept ourselves, we stop fighting with our own thoughts and feelings. Instead, we allow ourselves to exist as we are, which helps us live more peacefully.

Many people think self-acceptance means we have to love everything about ourselves all the time. But that is not exactly correct. Loving ourselves constantly can be wonderful, but self-acceptance also includes moments when we do not feel perfect or lovable. Sometimes we face anger, sadness, or insecurity, and those emotions can make us doubt our value. However, when we practice self-acceptance, we allow ourselves to have these emotions without believing they define our worth.

The Meaning of Self-Acceptance

Self-acceptance means looking at who we are right now and saying, "I am okay with me." It does not mean we cannot change. In fact, when we accept ourselves first, we often feel freer to grow, because we are no longer held back by shame.

For instance, imagine you are learning a new skill, like drawing. If you cannot accept your beginner drawings, you might feel embarrassed and give up. But with self-acceptance, you understand that you are allowed to be a beginner. You are allowed to make mistakes. As a result, you keep trying and eventually become better at drawing.

Key Aspects of Self-Acceptance

- **Honesty**: We need to be honest with ourselves about what we feel, think, and do. Hiding from our feelings or pretending to be someone else can hurt our progress.

- **Compassion**: Treating ourselves with understanding and kindness even when we stumble or fail.
- **Willingness to Grow**: Accepting ourselves does not mean we stop improving. It means we do not let shame or harsh self-judgment block us from learning and growing.

Why Self-Acceptance Matters

Think about how much time you spend worrying about what other people think of you. Or how often you criticize yourself for not being good enough, pretty enough, or smart enough. All these habits can limit your happiness and keep you trapped in a cycle of negativity. Self-acceptance allows you to break free from that cycle.

Once you stop attacking yourself for being "less than perfect," your mind becomes calmer. You start to notice the good traits you have. You see that you are capable of learning. You realize you can be kind to yourself without needing external approval.

Emotional Benefits

- **Reduced Stress**: Constant self-criticism causes stress and anxiety. Self-acceptance helps reduce this tension by replacing harsh self-talk with understanding and patience.
- **Improved Self-Esteem**: By seeing your worth in an honest and balanced way, you boost your self-esteem naturally.
- **More Resilience**: When you accept yourself, you can handle setbacks better. You know that mistakes do not make you worthless. They are just moments to learn from.

Practical Benefits

- **Better Relationships**: When you accept yourself, you are less likely to look to others for constant reassurance. This reduces pressure on your friendships and partnerships.
- **Improved Creativity**: Worrying about being judged often stifles creativity. But if you let yourself explore ideas, you open the door to new ways of thinking.

- **Clearer Decision-Making**: Instead of making decisions out of fear or guilt, you learn to make choices that align with your true self.

Common Blocks to Self-Acceptance

Self-acceptance can feel like a big mountain to climb. Why? Because many of us have old beliefs about not being good enough. These beliefs could stem from childhood experiences, relationships, or cultural pressures that teach us to measure our worth by things outside of us—like achievements or appearances.

Fear of Not Being Enough

One of the biggest reasons people struggle with self-acceptance is the fear that they are not sufficient. They worry that if they accept themselves, they might stay "flawed" forever. But self-acceptance is not about giving up on growth. It is about letting go of shame.

Comparison with Others

We often compare ourselves to others—friends, celebrities, social media personalities—and decide we do not measure up. This comparison trap can rob us of peace. When we compare ourselves to an unrealistic image, we end up feeling unhappy. Self-acceptance helps us refocus on our own journey, acknowledging that everyone has different strengths and weaknesses.

Negative Inner Voice

We all have an inner voice that talks to us throughout the day. If that voice is constantly negative, it can be tough to develop self-acceptance. For example, if your inner voice says, "I am stupid" every time you make a mistake, you will start to believe it, and acceptance will feel impossible.

Steps Towards Self-Acceptance

Learning to accept yourself is a journey. You do not snap your fingers and suddenly feel total peace with who you are. But if you take consistent steps, you can make real progress.

1. **Notice Your Feelings**: Pay attention to how you feel in different situations. Are there moments you feel especially harsh on yourself? Understanding these triggers is the first step.
2. **Challenge Negative Beliefs**: When you catch yourself thinking negatively about who you are, ask if that thought is actually true. Often, it is just an old belief, not a fact.
3. **Practice Self-Compassion**: When you fail or make mistakes, respond to yourself kindly. Imagine how you would talk to a friend going through the same situation.
4. **Seek Support**: Sometimes talking to a counselor, friend, or support group can help you break patterns of self-judgment.

Self-Acceptance vs. Self-Improvement

People often fear that accepting themselves means they will not be motivated to improve. Actually, self-improvement works best when it is built on a base of self-acceptance. If you accept who you are, you will feel less pressure and more clarity to set goals that truly reflect your needs and desires.

For example, let us say you want to get in better physical shape. If you begin your journey from a place of self-hatred—telling yourself you are unattractive or unworthy until you lose weight—you may end up quitting or feeling miserable. But if you start from acceptance, you are more likely to form healthy habits that you can maintain in the long run.

Real-Life Examples

Consider these real-life scenarios where self-acceptance plays a big role:

- **Changing Careers**: A person might want to switch careers but feels trapped by the fear of failure. With self-acceptance, they understand that it is okay to be new at something. They allow themselves to be a beginner without feeling ashamed.
- **Public Speaking**: If you have to give a speech and you are worried people will judge your performance, self-acceptance reminds you that it is okay to be nervous. You can still deliver your message even if your voice trembles a bit.

- **Appearance Insecurities**: Someone might always wear clothing to hide perceived flaws. With self-acceptance, they learn to dress in ways that feel comfortable rather than strictly trying to hide. Over time, this eases their worries about body image.

Small Ways to Start Practicing Self-Acceptance

1. **Write Down Compliments You Receive**: Often, we forget the good things people say about us. Keeping a small notebook of compliments can remind you that you have strengths others see.
2. **Celebrate Small Wins**: Did you cook a meal you have never tried before? That is a win. Did you get through a tough day at work? That is also a win. Recognizing these small victories teaches your mind to notice what you do right.
3. **Spend Time Alone**: Whether it is a quiet walk or simply taking a few moments to breathe, spending time alone can help you connect with your inner world. You become more aware of your thoughts and emotions, which is the first step toward acceptance.
4. **Focus on What You Can Control**: Understand the difference between what you can change and what you cannot. You can control your effort and how you treat yourself, but not every circumstance in your life. By focusing on what you can change, you avoid feeling helpless.

The Power of Telling Your Story

Sharing your personal story can help with self-acceptance. When you talk about your struggles and successes, you learn to see your journey as part of who you are. This does not mean you have to post your life story on social media. You might just share it with a close friend or write it in a private journal.

When we hide our experiences, we often feel shame. By bringing them to the light, we become more comfortable with ourselves and recognize we are not alone.

The Ongoing Journey

Self-acceptance is not a one-time event. It is more like a continuous process—sometimes you will feel you have made huge progress, and other times you may slip into old habits of self-doubt. That is normal. Life events, like a new job or a breakup, can bring new challenges to self-acceptance.

But remember, each time you pick yourself up and remind yourself that you are worthy, you strengthen your ability to accept yourself. Over time, you become more confident and peaceful.

Practice Exercise

- **Reflection Time**: Take five to ten minutes today to sit quietly. Close your eyes if it feels comfortable. Notice if any negative thoughts come up about yourself. Write down a few of those thoughts afterward. Then, write a gentle response to each. For example, if you think, "I am such a failure," write, "I am allowed to fail, and I can learn from this."

This simple exercise can teach you to challenge harmful beliefs and choose kinder thoughts instead.

Looking Ahead

In the next chapter, we will explore the roots of low self-worth and how it develops over time. Understanding where self-judgment begins can help us unravel it and build a solid foundation for deeper self-acceptance.

Remember, you do not have to be perfect to be worth acceptance. You are worth accepting right now, just as you are.

CHAPTER 2: THE ROOTS OF LOW SELF-WORTH

Low self-worth can show up in many ways. Some people feel it as a sense of emptiness or a belief that they do not deserve love and respect. Others feel it as shame or embarrassment about themselves. In order to practice self-acceptance, it is important to understand where these negative feelings come from. Once you see the causes, it becomes easier to tackle them.

Early Influences: Childhood and Environment

Childhood is a powerful time. We pick up lessons from our parents, siblings, teachers, and friends, often without realizing it. If a child is constantly criticized or made to feel that mistakes are unacceptable, they might grow up fearing that they are not good enough. Even well-meaning parents can sometimes send messages that cause low self-worth if they push a child too hard to achieve or behave in a certain way.

How Childhood Shapes Our Beliefs

- **Critical Households**: Growing up in a critical environment can make children view themselves negatively. For instance, if a child repeatedly hears, "You are never doing this right," they might believe they lack competence.
- **Overprotectiveness**: Overprotective guardians can unintentionally teach children that the world is dangerous and that they cannot handle challenges on their own. This can lead to low confidence.
- **Comparisons**: If a child is often compared to siblings or classmates, they may feel they are not meeting expectations, especially if the comparisons are harsh or frequent.

Societal Pressures

Even outside the home, many social forces can damage our sense of worth. Society can put people into "boxes" or categories, judging them by appearance, success, or financial status. Advertisements often show "perfect" lifestyles and bodies, making regular people feel inadequate.

Social media can add another layer of pressure, because it is easy to believe that everyone else is living a perfect life. We see filtered photos and polished videos, and compare them to our own messy reality. Over time, this can harm our self-esteem if we do not recognize that social media rarely shows the full story.

Toxic Relationships and Bullying

Some relationships can also harm our self-worth. If you have ever been in a toxic relationship—whether it is a romantic partner, a friend, or a coworker—you might have felt put down, manipulated, or ignored. When someone constantly treats you badly, it is normal to start believing their hurtful words.

Bullying is another factor, especially in childhood and teenage years. Constant bullying can stay with a person long after the bullying stops, leading them to feel small or unsafe even in new social settings.

Internalizing Mistakes and Failures

Everyone fails sometimes. That is part of being human. But if you have low self-worth, you might see failures not as temporary setbacks but as proof that you are a flawed person. You might think, "I failed at this, so I am a failure." This harmful way of thinking can become a cycle, where each small mistake feeds your negative view of yourself.

Breaking the Cycle

1. **Realize that failure is normal**: Remember that everyone fails at something. It is okay to learn from mistakes and move forward.
2. **Separate actions from self**: If you fail a test, it does not mean you are "stupid." It means you did not do well this time. You can study differently or seek help next time.
3. **Focus on growth**: Treat mistakes as lessons rather than proof of inadequacy.

Cultural and Community Factors

Some cultures place strong emphasis on certain values like family honor, academic success, or physical appearance. If a person does not meet these expectations, they might feel guilt or shame. Additionally, some communities have strict ideas about how people should act or what success means.

For example, in a community that places high value on formal education, a person who struggles in school might feel they are less worthy. Or in places where physical appearance is prized, those who look different might feel pressured to conform. Over time, these cultural messages can chip away at self-worth.

How Low Self-Worth Affects Daily Life

People with low self-worth often experience issues in many areas of life, such as:

- **Relationships**: They might struggle to stand up for themselves or set boundaries. They may stay in unhealthy relationships because they believe they do not deserve better.
- **Work and Career**: They might not apply for promotions or new opportunities, convinced they are not qualified even when they are.
- **Mental Health**: Low self-worth is linked to issues like depression, anxiety, and chronic stress.
- **Personal Growth**: People who feel unworthy might avoid exploring new hobbies or learning skills because they expect to fail.

Recognizing the Signs of Low Self-Worth

Sometimes, people do not realize they have low self-worth. They might simply think they are "being realistic" or "humble." But there is a difference between healthy humility and feeling inherently inadequate.

Common Signs

- **Harsh Self-Talk**: Constantly calling yourself names or putting yourself down in your mind.

- **Difficulty Accepting Compliments**: Feeling uncomfortable or disbelieving when someone says something nice about you.
- **Fear of Rejection**: Letting the fear of being rejected stop you from reaching out or trying new things.
- **People-Pleasing**: Always saying "yes" to others, even at your own expense, because you crave their approval.
- **Self-Sabotage**: Starting to do well at something but quitting or causing problems for yourself out of fear of success or the belief you do not deserve it.

Reframing Past Experiences

It is important to revisit old memories and see how they might be affecting your self-worth today. This does not mean we should blame everything on our past or stay stuck in it. Rather, we examine our history to understand where unhealthy thought patterns came from so we can change them.

Example: Overly Critical Parent

Let us say you had a parent who rarely praised your efforts. If you got an A minus on a test, they might say, "Why is this not an A plus?" As a child, you might have decided that nothing you do is ever good enough. As an adult, you may continue to chase perfection or harshly judge yourself when you fall short.

How to Heal

1. **Acknowledge the past**: Recognize the root cause. Understand that your parent's actions shaped your self-beliefs.
2. **Challenge those beliefs**: Remind yourself that you are not a child anymore and that you do not have to judge yourself by those old standards.
3. **Practice self-compassion**: When you achieve something, allow yourself to feel proud, even if it is not "perfect."

Embracing Our Personal Journey

Everyone's journey is different. Some people develop low self-worth from a single traumatic event, while others face a mix of smaller negative experiences that add up over time. Recognizing the different influences is the first step in freeing ourselves from them.

We can learn to see ourselves in a kinder light by reframing these life events. Maybe you had to grow up quickly because of family troubles, and that made you believe you were not allowed to make mistakes. With awareness, you can realize that your worth does not hinge on always being strong or perfect.

Creating a New Foundation

Low self-worth often sits on a shaky foundation of old beliefs and experiences. To build a better sense of self, we need to create a new foundation—one based on honesty, kindness, and a willingness to accept imperfection.

Practical Steps

- **Self-Reflection Journals**: Write about moments in your past that made you doubt your worth. Then write a more balanced view of each event.
- **Positive Role Models**: Seek out stories of people who overcame similar challenges or who demonstrate self-acceptance. Seeing how others have healed can inspire you.
- **Therapy or Counseling**: A mental health professional can guide you in untangling deep-rooted beliefs. This support can be very helpful if you feel overwhelmed.

Overcoming the "Should" Mindset

We often have "should" statements in our heads: "I should have done better," "I should be thinner," or "I should not show weakness." These "shoulds" can weigh us down, implying that there is only one acceptable way to be or feel.

Try replacing "should" with "could." Instead of "I should have done better," say, "I could try a different strategy next time." This small shift in language can encourage self-growth instead of piling on guilt.

The Role of Acceptance in Healing

When we understand that our low self-worth can come from a variety of experiences—family, culture, social pressure—our perspective changes. We realize many factors shaped us, and it is not because we truly are unworthy. This realization can spark hope.

Accepting Where We Are

Acceptance does not mean we like all the reasons our self-worth might be low. It means we stop trying to deny or hide them. By doing so, we give ourselves permission to heal. It is like opening a window in a dark room, letting some light in, and seeing what is really there.

Looking Beyond Blame

It can be tempting to blame parents or bullies for our struggles. While it is valid to acknowledge hurtful actions, staying stuck in blame can prevent growth. Low self-worth might have been influenced by those around us, but it is now our responsibility to fix how we see ourselves.

Taking ownership of our healing does not excuse harmful behavior from the past. Instead, it puts the power back in our hands. We decide how to move forward.

Reconnecting with Our Inner Voice

Earlier, we looked at how a negative inner voice can shape our self-image. The roots of that voice can come from our past—criticisms or judgments that we internalized. But we can gradually change that inner voice.

Steps to Reconnect

1. **Observe**: Throughout the day, notice what you say to yourself. Are you encouraging or critical?
2. **Question**: If the voice is harsh, ask, "Whose voice is this really?" Sometimes it is an echo from your past, not your own reasoning.

3. **Rewrite**: Replace harsh statements with a gentler or more balanced thought.

Building Healthier Relationships

If toxic relationships or bullying harmed your self-worth, you might need to build new, healthier connections. Seek people who treat you with respect and kindness, and who support your journey toward self-acceptance.

Sometimes this involves setting boundaries—learning to say no when people push your limits. It might mean reducing contact with people who constantly criticize you. Building healthier relationships is an important part of creating a supportive environment for your new, more positive self-view.

A Personal Reflection Exercise

Try this simple reflection to understand the roots of your own low self-worth:

1. **Quiet Moment**: Find a quiet space. Take a deep breath.
2. **Earliest Memory**: Think of a memory from childhood where you felt you were "not good enough." Write down what happened and how you felt.
3. **Adult Perspective**: Now read that memory and respond as an adult. Comfort your younger self. Write a message of reassurance, such as, "You were a child doing your best."
4. **Future Intention**: Finally, note one small thing you can do to remind yourself that you are worthy and growing, such as seeking out a supportive friend or practicing positive affirmations.

Conclusion: Moving Forward with Awareness

Realizing where our low self-worth comes from gives us awareness. We see that it does not appear out of thin air—we are shaped by family, culture, experiences, and our own thought patterns. This knowledge helps us break free.

Remember:

- You can honor your past without letting it define you.
- You can question old beliefs and replace them with more truthful ones.

- You can surround yourself with people and experiences that lift you up.

By moving forward with this awareness, you set the stage for the next steps in self-acceptance. In the upcoming chapters, we will dive deeper into specific tools for handling negative self-talk, nurturing our strengths, and developing a healthier relationship with ourselves.

CHAPTER 3: FACING NEGATIVE SELF-TALK

Negative self-talk is the inner voice that criticizes you. It might call you names, highlight your flaws, or fill your mind with fear. This voice does not speak the full truth about who you are, but it often feels powerful. Sometimes it whispers, sometimes it shouts. It can stop you from trying new things, or fill your days with worry. Learning to face negative self-talk is an important step in self-acceptance because it helps clear the path for a kinder and more supportive relationship with yourself.

Recognizing Negative Self-Talk

Many people do not notice their negative self-talk. The voice can be so familiar that you think it is normal or even true. But negative self-talk usually carries a harsh tone and blows things out of proportion. Here are some ways it might appear:

1. **Name-Calling in Your Mind**: For example, if you drop a glass and it breaks, do you instantly think, "I am so stupid" or "I always mess up"?
2. **Assuming the Worst**: You might think, "Nobody will like me," or "I will fail, so why even try?"
3. **Blaming Yourself for Everything**: If something goes wrong, do you instantly believe it is all your fault?

Notice that negative self-talk often uses sweeping language like *always* or *never*. It does not allow for the idea that sometimes things go right or that you do have strengths.

Why Negative Self-Talk Forms

This inner critic does not appear from nowhere. It usually has roots in past experiences, lessons we picked up from our environment, or even cultural messages that tell us we are not enough.

- **Past Criticism**: Harsh words from parents, teachers, or peers in childhood can settle into our mind and become our own internal voice.
- **Fear of Failure**: Sometimes we criticize ourselves to avoid disappointment. We think that if we do not get our hopes up, we will not be let down.
- **Perfectionism**: If you believe you must always perform at your best, any sign of imperfection can trigger the negative voice.

Understanding why negative self-talk forms can help you see it as a learned response rather than an unchangeable fact of life.

The Effects of Negative Self-Talk

Negative self-talk can affect almost every part of your life. It can make you feel anxious, reduce your motivation, and even hurt your relationships with others. If you believe you are not worthy or able to succeed, you might avoid challenges that would help you grow. You might also push away people who try to support you, because you do not trust that they care about you for who you are.

Emotional Drain

Hearing negative thoughts day in and day out can drain your emotional energy. You might feel tired or sad without fully understanding why. Over time, this can turn into ongoing stress or even depression. When your own mind seems to be against you, it is hard to find peace.

Blocks to Personal Growth

Imagine you want to learn a new skill, like dancing. If your mind constantly tells you that you look silly or that you will never be good enough, it is easy to give up before you begin. Negative self-talk acts like a chain that holds you back from trying, failing, and improving. It stops you from seeing the path forward, so you stay still.

Impact on Relationships

When you have a harsh inner critic, it might make you sensitive to any hint of criticism from others. You might assume people are judging you, even if they are not. Or you may become defensive to protect yourself. On the other hand, some people become people-pleasers, bending over backward to avoid disapproval, because their own mind is already so critical.

Strategies to Challenge Negative Self-Talk

Recognizing negative self-talk is one thing. Changing it is another. The good news is that our minds are flexible. We can train ourselves to speak more kindly. This does not mean forcing ourselves to think everything is perfect, but it does mean finding a balance.

Step 1: Listen and Identify

The first step is to listen carefully to the words you say to yourself. Spend a few days writing down your negative thoughts in a small notebook or on your phone. Even just noting a phrase like, "I messed up again. I am hopeless," can help you see how often this inner critic appears.

Step 2: Question the Negative Beliefs

When you see a negative thought, ask yourself if it is based on facts or fear. Often, you will find it is not as solid as it seems. For example, if you think, "I am always messing up," ask yourself: "Is that actually true? Am I truly messing up all the time? What about the times I succeed?"

Step 3: Replace with Balanced Thoughts

The goal is not blind positivity or telling yourself things you do not believe. Instead, try to replace an extreme negative statement with a more balanced one. For instance, "I made a mistake this time, but that does not mean I always fail." This approach respects reality while reducing unfair self-criticism.

Step 4: Practice Self-Compassion

Self-compassion means treating yourself with the same kindness you would show a friend. When you catch negative self-talk, imagine that a close friend spoke those words about themselves. How would you respond to them? Most likely, you would be patient, supportive, and understanding. Offer that same gentle tone to yourself.

Reframing Mistakes

One of the most common triggers for negative self-talk is making mistakes. But mistakes are natural. Everyone makes them. They are a normal part of growth. Instead of seeing a mistake as proof of unworthiness, recognize that it is a chance to learn. Even experts in any field made errors along the way.

- **Reflect**: Ask, "What can I learn from this error?"
- **Act**: Try a new approach next time.
- **Move Forward**: Do not replay the failure repeatedly in your mind.

Separating the Inner Critic from Reality

Sometimes it helps to think of the negative voice as a separate character rather than your true self. You can even give it a silly name if that helps you distance yourself from it. When you hear that voice say, "You will never be good at this," you can respond, "Thanks for your concern, but I am going to try anyway."

This method reminds you that negative self-talk is not your ultimate guide. It is just one perspective, often formed by fear or past conditioning.

The Role of Encouraging Self-Talk

Just as harmful as negative self-talk can be, encouraging self-talk can be a powerful tool for healing and motivation. Imagine if, when you felt unsure, your mind said, "You have done hard things before, you can do this too." Over time, these words can become a supportive habit that helps you keep going.

How to Cultivate Encouraging Thoughts

1. **Use Reminders**: Write short, positive phrases on notes and stick them where you will see them. For example, on your mirror you might write, "I am growing every day."
2. **Celebrate Small Wins**: When you finish a task—big or small—allow yourself to feel happy about it. This teaches your mind to recognize achievements rather than only errors.
3. **Practice Gratitude**: Think of a few things you are grateful for each day. Gratitude can shift your focus from what is lacking to what you do have.

Negative Self-Talk and Stress

Negative thoughts can fuel stress. If your mind is always in a battle—reminding you of worries, scolding you for mistakes—you never feel fully at ease. Your body might respond with tension in your muscles, headaches, or trouble sleeping. Stress from negative self-talk can also make it hard to concentrate, which then causes more anxiety about messing up. It is a cycle that feeds on itself.

Breaking the Cycle

Breaking the cycle starts with awareness. When you notice you are entering a spiral of negative thoughts, pause. Take a slow, deep breath. You can even step away from the situation for a moment. That short break gives you time to question the negative thinking and remind yourself that you do not have to believe it.

Learning from Setbacks

Sometimes, no matter how much we try to stay positive, life throws us obstacles. We might lose a job, fail an exam, or face rejection. At these times, negative self-talk can become louder because we think the setback proves we are not good enough. But setbacks do not have to confirm negative beliefs. They can be opportunities to build resilience.

- **Focus on What You Can Control**: You cannot always change the outcome, but you can change your approach to it.
- **Reach Out for Support**: Talk to a friend, counselor, or family member. Sharing your feelings can help you see the situation in a new way.
- **Give Yourself Time**: Healing from disappointment does not happen overnight. Be patient with yourself.

The Difference Between Criticism and Self-Reflection

Some people worry that if they stop negative self-talk, they will not recognize areas where they need to improve. But there is a difference between healthy self-reflection and harsh criticism. Healthy self-reflection is honest but not cruel. It focuses on growth rather than punishing yourself.

Example of Healthy Self-Reflection

- "I notice I have been procrastinating on my project. Maybe I am scared of failing. I can plan a schedule and break the project into smaller tasks to manage my fear."

This type of reflection acknowledges a challenge, looks for the reason behind it, and proposes a solution. There is no attack on your worth as a person.

Building a Support System

Overcoming negative self-talk is easier when you have a support system. Friends, family members, support groups, or counselors can help you see yourself more clearly. Sometimes we need an external voice to remind us of our strengths.

Talking About Your Inner Critic

It can feel vulnerable to share that you have a harsh inner voice. But opening up about it can be healing. You might discover that many people have a similar struggle. Even just saying, "I am working on changing the way I talk to myself," can make you feel less alone.

Practical Exercises for Facing Negative Self-Talk

Here are a few actions you can try:

1. **Daily Check-In**: At the end of each day, write down one instance of negative self-talk you caught. Then rewrite it in a more balanced way.
2. **Mindful Breathing**: When your thoughts become too loud, focus on your breath for 30 seconds. Inhale slowly, then exhale. This can help reset your mind.
3. **Visualize a Compassionate Mentor**: Imagine someone you admire telling you kind and encouraging words. This could be a teacher, a grandparent,

or even a character from a movie. Let their imagined voice guide you to a gentler mindset.

Overcoming the Fear of Positive Self-Talk

For some people, positive or encouraging self-talk feels awkward or fake, especially if they have been used to the opposite for a long time. They might think, "If I tell myself nice things, I will just be lying." But in truth, you are not lying when you say something encouraging. You are choosing to see that your worth is not limited to your flaws.

Practice takes time. Start by finding a short sentence you can believe, such as, "I am allowed to make mistakes," or, "I am a person learning each day." Over time, you can build on that foundation.

Changing the Tone of Your Inner Dialogue

An effective way to shift your self-talk is to pay attention not just to what you say but *how* you say it in your mind. Do you speak to yourself in a harsh tone or a gentle tone? This might sound a bit abstract, but we all have a certain "voice" in our heads. Try softening that voice. When you talk to yourself internally, imagine you are speaking to someone you truly care about.

When Negative Self-Talk Persists

Even after practicing these strategies, there will be days when negative self-talk sneaks in. That is normal. Habits do not vanish overnight. The key is to be patient and not be hard on yourself for having negative thoughts. Instead of saying, "I failed at positive thinking," remind yourself, "It takes time to form new mental habits, and every step matters."

Personal Reflection: Your Journey with Negative Self-Talk

Take a moment to think about your earliest memory of self-criticism. Can you recall a time in your life when you first felt that stinging voice telling you that you were not good enough? Maybe it was after a poor grade, a fight with a friend, or a comment from a parent. Write that memory down, along with the words you told yourself.

Then ask: "Is that view still accurate, or is it just an echo from the past?" Give yourself permission to see that event from a more balanced viewpoint. You were younger then, with less experience. Now, you know more, and you can treat yourself more fairly.

The Power of Self-Forgiveness

One reason negative self-talk lingers is because of guilt or shame over past actions. Maybe you regret something you said to a loved one, or a decision you made that hurt you or others. While it is important to learn from mistakes, carrying endless self-blame hurts your ability to accept yourself today.

Self-forgiveness does not mean you pretend the mistake did not happen. It means you acknowledge it, do what you can to make amends, and then allow yourself to move on. Holding onto blame forever does not fix anything; it simply feeds that harsh inner critic.

Looking Forward

Facing negative self-talk is a key part of building self-acceptance. When you learn to spot harmful thoughts, question them, and replace them with fairer statements, you open the door to greater peace. You also free yourself to try new things and build stronger connections with others. It takes dedication, but each small step helps you form a more caring and supportive inner world.

In the next chapter, we will explore the importance of embracing our flaws—seeing them not as reasons for shame but as natural parts of being human. Understanding this can further quiet that negative voice, helping us stand confidently, even with our imperfections.

CHAPTER 4: EMBRACING OUR FLAWS

We all have flaws. They can be physical, emotional, or behavioral. Some flaws are obvious to us, while others only show up in certain situations. In many cultures, people try hard to hide their flaws because they worry about being judged. But true self-acceptance involves not only tolerating our imperfections but also making peace with them. When we embrace our flaws, we stop wasting energy on hiding what we consider wrong with us. Instead, we learn that these imperfections are part of our humanity.

What Does It Mean to Embrace Our Flaws?

Embracing our flaws does not mean we have to love them or stop trying to grow. It simply means recognizing that flaws are normal and do not erase our worth. For example, if you are forgetful, embracing that flaw means you accept that sometimes you will forget things. You then look for ways to manage it—like using reminders—without feeling ashamed or viewing it as a sign of personal failure.

Why We Struggle with Accepting Flaws

A big reason we struggle with flaws is that society often values perfection. We see pictures of people who seem flawless, or we read stories of high-achievers who seem to never make mistakes. This can create an unrealistic standard. In reality, everyone has something they consider a flaw.

- **Fear of Rejection**: Many people worry that if they show their flaws, others will reject them.
- **Perfectionism**: We may feel we should always get things right, so any mistake becomes a source of shame.
- **Cultural Expectations**: Some societies or families have strict norms about how a person should look or act, making it hard to accept anything that falls outside of those norms.

The Danger of Trying to Hide Flaws

When we try to hide our flaws at all costs, we create stress for ourselves. We might avoid situations where our weaknesses could be revealed, which can limit our experiences. For instance, if someone believes they are bad at public speaking, they might refuse opportunities to speak in front of others—even if doing so would help them grow or succeed at work. This avoidance can shrink our world and keep us from discovering what we are truly capable of.

Additionally, hiding flaws makes it hard to form genuine connections with others. We are constantly worried about being "found out." True closeness with others often comes from shared vulnerability—when people feel safe to reveal their real selves, flaws included.

Finding Acceptance in Imperfection

It can be helpful to think of flaws as something that makes us unique. Imagine a person with a small gap between their teeth, which they used to hate. One day, they realize this gap sets them apart and can even be seen as charming. Embracing that physical flaw becomes a way to celebrate uniqueness rather than be ashamed.

Not all flaws are simply physical quirks. Some are deeper habits or character traits. If you have a quick temper, for example, embracing it means understanding that you have a tendency to get angry. You then work on managing it better, but you stop feeling like you must pretend you are always calm.

Learning from Our Flaws

Flaws can also teach us valuable lessons. A person who struggles with patience might learn how to slow down and listen carefully. A person who is shy might discover the importance of small, meaningful friendships rather than numerous casual ones. By looking at our flaws with curiosity instead of shame, we can uncover strengths that come from them.

Example: Turning a Flaw into Strength

Let us say you are overly cautious. You might take extra time to make decisions, which some see as a flaw because it slows you down. But that same cautious nature can protect you from rushing into bad choices. Embracing your careful side means you acknowledge that yes, you can be slow in certain moments, but it also helps you be thorough.

Practical Steps to Embrace Your Flaws

Step 1: Identify Your Flaws

Make a list of traits you consider flaws. Write them down honestly, but do not judge yourself harshly. You are simply noting what you see. For example, you might write: "Impatient when waiting in line, scared to speak up in groups, prone to daydreaming when I should be working."

Step 2: Reflect on Each Flaw

Spend time understanding each flaw. Ask yourself questions like:

- "Where did this flaw come from?"
- "Is it always negative, or does it sometimes help me?"
- "How do I feel when I try to hide it?"

Step 3: Find Ways to Manage (If Needed)

Some flaws, like a tendency to be late, may require practical solutions (like setting multiple alarms or planning ahead). Other flaws, like being sensitive to criticism, might call for emotional tools (like learning to breathe through anxiety or seeking a friend's support). The main point is to manage your flaw without feeling shame.

Step 4: Look for Silver Linings

Many flaws have a flip side that can be positive. If you are sensitive, you might also be empathetic toward others' feelings. If you are stubborn, you might also be persistent in chasing your goals. Recognizing these positives helps you see that a flaw can be a strength in the right setting.

Self-Talk Around Flaws

We often have harsh self-talk around our flaws. We might say, "I am an idiot," or "I am ugly," or "I always do this wrong." To embrace flaws, we need to change that language. Instead of saying, "I am an idiot for forgetting my keys," say, "I forgot my keys today. Let me figure out a better system so I will remember next time." This shift moves away from name-calling and toward problem-solving.

Modeling Self-Acceptance for Others

When we embrace our own flaws, we also give permission for others to do the same. This can improve relationships. For instance, if you openly admit, "I tend to be messy, but I am working on keeping my space organized," friends or family may feel more comfortable sharing their own struggles. Openness can create a space of mutual understanding and acceptance.

Flaws and Personal Boundaries

Embracing your flaws does not mean you have to accept disrespect from others. If someone constantly teases you or belittles you for a flaw, it is okay to set a boundary. You can be honest about your imperfection but still stand up for how you should be treated. For example, you might say, "Yes, I know I am forgetful, but I would appreciate if you did not call me lazy or useless because of it."

Setting boundaries can protect your sense of worth and show that embracing a flaw does not equal tolerating hurtful behavior.

Overcoming Shame

Flaws often create shame if we believe they make us "less than" others. But shame is not a healthy emotion when it comes to imperfections. It does not help us grow, it just makes us feel small. One approach to overcoming shame is to talk about your flaw with someone you trust. Hearing them respond with kindness can chip away at the shame you feel.

- **Example**: You might say, "I have always felt really insecure about how I freeze up in social gatherings." A friend might reply, "I freeze up too sometimes. It is normal to feel that way." This can help you see you are not alone in your flaw.

Letting Go of Comparisons

We tend to compare our flaws to someone else's strengths. You might see a friend who is very organized and think, "Why can't I be that organized?" But remember, everyone has a different set of flaws and strengths. Comparing yourself to someone else is rarely helpful because you do not see the full picture of their life. They may admire qualities in you that you are not even aware of.

Embracing Flaws and Personal Growth

There is a common misunderstanding that if you accept your flaws, you will not want to improve. However, embracing your flaws actually reduces the shame that keeps you stuck. Without shame, you are freer to take a good look at yourself and see where you can grow. You do not have to pretend you have no flaws; you simply acknowledge them without letting them define your entire worth.

Example of Growth Through Acceptance

If you have trouble staying focused, embracing that fact means you admit, "I can get distracted easily." From there, you might create a more structured routine or learn techniques to improve concentration. You do not waste time beating yourself up or trying to hide it. Instead, you move forward with a sense of calm responsibility.

Balancing Flaws with Realistic Expectations

While it is good to accept we are flawed, it is also important to set realistic expectations for ourselves. We should not use our flaws as excuses to stop trying or to justify harmful behavior. For example, if someone has a short temper, they can say, "I accept I have a quick temper, but I will work on healthy ways to express anger so I do not hurt those around me."

This balance allows for honesty about who we are and a commitment to being the best version of ourselves.

Building Compassionate Self-Awareness

Embracing flaws becomes easier when you develop a compassionate self-awareness. That means you understand your strengths and weaknesses, but you hold them in kindness rather than judgment. When you notice a flaw surfacing—like you are about to lose your temper—you can take a breath and say, "Okay, here is that temper again. I know it is part of me, but I also know I can handle it better."

Appreciating Flaws in Others

If you become more at peace with your own flaws, you might also find yourself being kinder toward others' imperfections. Instead of judging a coworker for always being late, you might think, "I know how it feels to struggle with time management." This understanding can create more harmony in your relationships. It also encourages a mutual sense of acceptance where everyone can show up as their real selves.

A Personal Exercise: Flaw Appreciation

Take a moment to write down one flaw you have never liked. Then ask yourself if there is any benefit or positive side to it. Maybe the flaw of being "overly emotional" makes you a more caring friend. Maybe a tendency to speak bluntly helps you be honest. Write down one or two ways this flaw has shaped you in a helpful way. This does not mean ignoring the challenges it brings, only that you recognize it might have value too.

Moving Away from Flaw-Focused Mindsets

Sometimes, we can get stuck focusing on our flaws as if they define us. But remember, you are more than your flaws. You have strengths, talents, hopes, and dreams. While it is good to acknowledge imperfections, do not let them overshadow the other parts of who you are. Think of your flaws as just one aspect of your full identity.

Living Authentically

When you embrace your flaws, you begin to live a more authentic life. You no longer have to pretend or hide major parts of yourself. This honesty can be refreshing and can inspire people around you. You may also find that you have more energy for creative pursuits and meaningful connections, because you are not wasting mental space worrying about looking perfect.

Conclusion: The Beauty of Imperfection

Embracing our flaws is an ongoing process. Some days, you might feel at peace with your imperfections; on other days, you might fall back into self-criticism. That is normal. What matters is that you keep reminding yourself that flaws are part of the human experience. They do not reduce your worth or make you unlovable.

By making peace with your flaws, you take a big step toward self-acceptance. You show yourself that you deserve kindness no matter what, and that you can continue to grow without punishing yourself for not being perfect. In the upcoming chapters, we will look at new ways to build a healthier inner dialogue and move through life with more confidence and peace.

Remember:

- You are allowed to be imperfect.
- You can accept yourself as you are and still work on the parts you want to change.
- Your flaws do not define you; they are simply part of your whole, wonderful self.

CHAPTER 5: BUILDING A POSITIVE INNER VOICE

In the previous chapters, we explored negative self-talk and learned about embracing our flaws. Now, it is time to take a more active step toward creating a healthier mental environment by building a positive inner voice. This voice acts like a kind, gentle companion inside your head. It can reassure you when you are stressed, encourage you when you feel unsure, and remind you of your value when life is tough. A positive inner voice does not mean you must ignore reality or pretend everything is perfect. Rather, it is about learning to talk to yourself in a manner that helps you thrive.

Understanding the Power of a Positive Inner Voice

A positive inner voice guides you like a supportive friend. Imagine a buddy who cheers you on, points out your progress, and helps you see solutions instead of dwelling on problems. That is what a positive inner voice can do. It is not about lying to yourself or dismissing challenges; it is about responding to those challenges with belief in your ability to handle them.

When your mind is filled with kindness rather than constant doubt, you become more open to new experiences. You might find yourself taking healthy risks, speaking up in groups, or trying out new hobbies. Instead of hearing, "I will mess up anyway," you hear, "Let's give it a shot and see what happens."

Why a Positive Inner Voice Matters

1. **Encouragement**: When you feel uncertain, your inner voice can say, "Keep going—you have faced hard things before and came through."
2. **Emotional Support**: On rough days, it can help calm your worries by focusing on hope, resilience, or whatever strengths you hold.
3. **Healthier Self-Esteem**: Over time, kind self-talk builds self-respect. You begin to see yourself as someone worthy of care and compassion.

How to Begin Shifting Your Inner Dialogue

Moving from a harsh inner critic to a more supportive voice takes practice. It is not an overnight change. You may find yourself slipping back into old, negative patterns. That is okay. Each time you notice negative self-talk, see it as an opportunity to introduce a more balanced, helpful thought.

Step 1: Pay Attention

Your first step is to pay closer attention to the words you say to yourself daily. This might involve writing in a journal or taking short notes on your phone whenever you catch a negative or critical thought. You cannot change what you do not see.

Step 2: Question the Negativity

As soon as you spot a harsh thought, ask, "Is this really true? Am I jumping to the worst conclusion?" Often, negative self-talk is based on fear or old habits rather than facts. If you catch yourself thinking, "I cannot do anything right," pause and see if that is truly correct. More likely, you have done many things right—but one failure or mistake is making you forget your successes.

Step 3: Introduce a Kinder Response

After you question a negative thought, come up with a kinder alternative. This does not mean you ignore any real problems. It means you respond to them in a supportive way. For example, if you failed at something, a kinder response might be, "I did not do well this time, but I can learn from it. I will try a new strategy or ask for help."

Finding the Tone That Feels Right

Some people find it easy to talk to themselves like they would to a close friend. Others feel awkward at first. If saying things like, "I love myself" feels unnatural, start with more neutral statements like, "I am trying my best," or, "I respect my efforts." Over time, as you become more comfortable, you can adjust your words to be more encouraging or affectionate.

Example Tones

- **Gentle Teacher**: "Let's see what we can learn from this challenge."
- **Compassionate Friend**: "It's okay to feel upset sometimes. I'm here for you."
- **Encouraging Coach**: "You got this. You have handled bigger things before."

Finding a tone that resonates with you makes it easier to stick with positive self-talk in the long run.

Overcoming Barriers to a Positive Inner Voice

Even if you want a more encouraging mindset, you might run into obstacles. You could have old beliefs that say you do not deserve kindness. Or perhaps you grew up in an environment where compliments and warmth were rare, so positivity feels foreign. These barriers can be overcome with consistent effort and self-awareness.

Recognizing Self-Sabotage

Self-sabotage is when you undermine your own progress. Sometimes, if a kind thought arises, you might immediately dismiss it as "corny" or "not true." This resistance often comes from fear—fear that embracing hope will lead to disappointment, or fear that being kind to yourself is "weak." Recognizing these moments helps you push through and remind yourself that nurturing a positive mindset is both healthy and brave.

Handling Setbacks

When life throws obstacles your way—like an unexpected failure, rejection, or loss—your old negative thoughts might get louder. You might wonder if being positive is "pointless." But these are exactly the times when a supportive inner voice matters most. It helps you cope with the setback by maintaining hope and reminding you of your ability to overcome hardships.

Practical Methods to Strengthen a Positive Voice

1. **Write Positive Notes**: Place small notes or sticky papers around your home with simple, encouraging phrases. For example: "You are doing a good job," or "It's okay to take it one step at a time."
2. **Record Affirmations**: If you are comfortable with it, record yourself saying positive statements. Listen to them when you feel doubt creeping in.
3. **Visualize Success**: Take a minute to imagine yourself completing a challenge successfully. Focus on how you would feel and what your supportive voice might say to keep you motivated.
4. **Celebrate Small Wins**: Each time you do something good—whether it is finishing a book, cleaning a room, or making a tough phone call—give yourself an internal pat on the back. These small acknowledgments add up and help your mind lean toward positivity.

Using Humor to Defuse Negativity

Sometimes, humor can be a powerful ally against negative self-talk. When you catch your mind spiraling into gloom, you might imagine a silly voice or cartoon character speaking those harsh words. It can make the negative thought seem less intimidating and more ridiculous. By reducing its severity, you create emotional space for a kinder thought to come in.

The Connection Between Positive Self-Talk and Confidence

Confidence often stems from trusting your own ability and worthiness. A positive inner voice reminds you that you have strengths—even if you have not yet developed all the skills you want. It encourages you to try, to fail without shame, and to keep going until you improve. Over time, as you see that you can tackle challenges, your confidence grows. The cycle continues: more confidence fuels more positive thinking, which then makes you feel even more capable.

A Quick Confidence Exercise

- Think of something you do fairly well, like cooking a certain dish, giving advice, or organizing your desk.
- Write down two to three sentences praising yourself for that ability. For example: "I make a delicious pasta. I love how I can combine flavors. My friends always enjoy my cooking."
- Read those lines out loud. Notice how you feel when you give yourself genuine praise.

This small exercise teaches your mind that it is okay and even beneficial to acknowledge the good in you.

Balancing Realism and Optimism

A positive inner voice does not ignore real problems. If you are struggling with finances, it would not help to say, "Everything is fine!" while ignoring late bills. Instead, you might acknowledge the reality—"I'm facing a tough time financially right now"—and then add a supportive statement: "I can look for new opportunities or budgeting tips to improve my situation. I believe I can find a solution." This approach maintains hope without losing touch with facts.

Building Positivity in Different Areas of Life

A supportive inner voice can apply to many areas:

- **Work or School**: Instead of saying, "I will never understand this assignment," try, "This assignment is challenging, but I can tackle it step by step."
- **Relationships**: If you fear asking for help, remind yourself, "People who care about me will want to support me when I need it."
- **Personal Goals**: Rather than "I'm too out of shape to start exercising," think, "I can start with small steps, like a short walk, and build up from there."

Creating a Positive Environment

Your inner voice can grow stronger if you also build a more encouraging environment around you. Spend time with people who uplift you and treat you kindly. Engage in activities that inspire you rather than activities that drain your confidence. Even the music, shows, and social media you consume can affect your mindset. If something consistently fuels negative thoughts, it might be time to reduce its presence in your life.

Setting Boundaries

Sometimes, you might have to set boundaries with people who constantly criticize you or belittle your efforts. This does not mean you must cut them off entirely (unless the relationship is truly harmful), but it could mean limiting your time with them or letting them know how their words affect you. Standing up for yourself in this way reinforces your own sense of worth.

Growth Through Positive Challenges

As your positive inner voice strengthens, you can use it to tackle new challenges. Maybe you sign up for a class you have always wanted to take or volunteer for a project at work. These challenges become opportunities to build your self-belief. Each time you accomplish something you thought you could not do, your mind learns that you are more capable than the negative voice once claimed.

When Positivity Feels Forced

It is normal to have moments where positivity feels forced or fake. Maybe you are in a really tough spot—facing illness, loss, or heartbreak. In such cases, it is okay to feel sad or worried. A healthy positive inner voice does not tell you to smile when your heart is hurting. Instead, it might say, "This is painful, and it's okay to feel upset. You're still strong, and you will find a way through this in time." That type of supportive honesty respects your feelings while still offering hope.

The Long-Term Impact of a Supportive Inner Voice

Over weeks and months of practicing kinder self-talk, you may notice that you are less anxious in everyday situations. You might feel more patient with yourself when you make errors. You begin to trust your ability to figure things out. While life will always have ups and downs, a positive inner voice can make those downs less overwhelming and the ups even more fulfilling.

Encouraging Others

As you get better at encouraging yourself, you might also start encouraging the people around you. When you hear a friend say something harsh about themselves, you can gently challenge that thought. By sharing your journey, you help others see the value of kinder self-talk, too.

Final Thoughts on Building a Positive Inner Voice

Building a positive inner voice is a lifelong process. As you gain new experiences, your self-talk may shift to match your growth. Be patient with this journey. If you slip back into negative patterns, do not be harsh on yourself—that only feeds the negativity. Instead, remind yourself that change is rarely linear, and every small effort counts.

A supportive inner voice lays a strong foundation for self-acceptance and inner peace. It helps you recognize your worth, even when life is not going perfectly. In the next chapter, we will look at how to overcome self-doubt and fear, two common hurdles that can shake our confidence and keep us from hearing that positive voice. Learning to face doubt and fear with courage will further strengthen your path toward true self-acceptance.

CHAPTER 6: OVERCOMING SELF-DOUBT AND FEAR

Self-doubt and fear can feel overwhelming. They can whisper in your ear, telling you that you are not ready, not good enough, or bound to fail. If you listen to these doubts for too long, you might never step out of your comfort zone. You could miss out on chances to learn, grow, and experience life more fully. In this chapter, we will explore practical ways to face self-doubt and fear so they do not hold you back from developing deeper self-acceptance and confidence.

Understanding Self-Doubt

Self-doubt is the feeling that you do not have what it takes to achieve a goal, solve a problem, or handle a situation. It might show up as a nagging voice that questions everything you do, or a deep worry that other people are better or more deserving. Like negative self-talk, self-doubt is often rooted in past experiences or comments from others that made you question your abilities.

The Effects of Self-Doubt

- **Paralysis by Analysis**: You might overthink simple decisions or spend excessive time weighing pros and cons, fearful of making a mistake.
- **Missed Opportunities**: If you always doubt yourself, you might avoid taking on challenges, missing out on learning and growth.
- **Strained Relationships**: Self-doubt can cause you to seek constant reassurance from friends or family, which can put stress on those relationships.

Recognizing Fear as a Natural Emotion

Fear is a basic human emotion designed to keep us safe from danger. However, fear can become overwhelming when it appears in situations that are not truly harmful. For example, you might feel fear at the idea of speaking in public or changing jobs, even though these activities are not life-threatening.

Healthy vs. Excessive Fear

- **Healthy Fear**: Helps you stay cautious, like avoiding walking too close to a high ledge.
- **Excessive Fear**: Stops you from trying safe new experiences or pursuing meaningful goals due to imagined worst-case scenarios.

When fear grows too large, it can keep you locked in place and feed into self-doubt.

Strategies to Overcome Self-Doubt

1. Gather Evidence of Your Capabilities

One way to fight self-doubt is to look back at what you have accomplished in the past. Make a list of times you succeeded at something challenging—even small victories count. By seeing real proof of your abilities, it becomes harder for doubt to convince you that you cannot do anything right.

Example

- You taught yourself a new hobby.
- You managed a tough situation at work.
- You reached out for help when you needed it.

Each of these actions shows resourcefulness, bravery, or growth. Use them as reminders that you have handled difficulties before and can do so again.

2. Challenge Perfectionism

Sometimes self-doubt comes from perfectionism—the belief that you must do everything flawlessly. But perfection is not realistic. Even experts make mistakes. Lowering the pressure to be perfect can help you see that you can try, fail, and keep going anyway. That sense of resilience is more valuable than never making mistakes.

3. Practice "What If" Scenarios in a Healthy Way

Self-doubt often thrives on negative "what if" questions, like: "What if I fail horribly?" or "What if everyone laughs at me?" Try flipping those thoughts around: "What if I learn something new?" or "What if this leads to an amazing opportunity?" Shifting to more hopeful "what ifs" can make a difference in how you approach unfamiliar tasks.

4. Talk to Someone You Trust

Sharing your doubts with a friend, family member, or counselor can help you see them more objectively. Often, another person can remind you of your strengths or point out flaws in your negative assumptions. This outside perspective can break the loop of constant self-questioning and help you gain confidence.

Facing Fear in a Constructive Way

1. Identify Your Specific Fears

Take time to define your fear clearly. Are you afraid of failure? Rejection? Embarrassment? Once you know exactly what you fear, you can address it directly. For instance, if you are afraid of public speaking, the specific fear might be "I will forget my lines and look foolish." Then you can plan ways to handle that possibility, such as writing note cards or practicing in front of a friend.

2. Use Gradual Exposure

Gradual exposure means facing your fear in small, manageable steps. If you fear speaking in public, you might start by practicing a short talk alone in your room. Then try it in front of one friend. Later, join a small group that practices public speaking. Each step helps you see that you can handle the challenge, reducing fear's power.

3. Visualize Success

Take a moment to sit quietly and imagine yourself successfully doing the thing you fear. Try to involve your senses—picture the room you are in, feel the emotions of confidence and relief when you do well. Visualization helps your brain see success as possible. Even though it is not the same as real experience, it can lower the emotional barrier that fear puts up.

4. Reward Yourself

Every time you do something that scares you—even if it is a small step—reward yourself. The reward can be a simple pat on the back, a tasty treat, or doing something you love. This positive reinforcement trains your mind to see facing fear as something beneficial rather than threatening.

Learning from Failure and Setbacks

Fear of failure is a major cause of self-doubt. But failure is not the end; it is part of any journey worth taking. When you see failure as a teacher rather than a punishment, you can overcome the dread of trying. Ask yourself: "What does this setback teach me?" Maybe it tells you to prepare better, seek advice, or try a different tactic. By embracing the lessons, you turn a disappointing moment into a stepping-stone for growth.

The Role of Self-Compassion in Facing Doubt and Fear

Self-compassion is vital when dealing with doubt and fear. If you judge yourself harshly for feeling scared, you add more pressure to an already stressful situation. Instead, treat yourself with patience and understanding. Accept that you are human and that fear is natural. Self-compassion can help you bounce back faster if things do not go as planned, because you do not waste energy beating yourself up.

A Quick Self-Compassion Exercise

- Close your eyes and take a deep breath.
- Remember a time you felt scared or doubted your ability.
- Gently place a hand on your chest (or anywhere it feels comfortable).
- Tell yourself, "It's okay to be worried. I'm here for me. I care about my well-being."

This exercise can calm your body and mind, making it easier to handle the fear without letting it consume you.

Building Resilience Against Future Doubts

Self-doubt and fear will likely appear again in your life, no matter how much you grow. But resilience means you can bounce back faster each time. Think of resilience like a muscle—you strengthen it every time you face a challenge, take a risk, or recover from failure. Over time, you gain faith in your own ability to adapt.

Habits That Encourage Resilience

- **Regular Reflection**: Spend a few minutes each day or week reviewing what you did well and what you learned.
- **Healthy Lifestyle**: Adequate sleep, balanced eating, and exercise can boost your mood and energy, making it easier to face challenges.
- **Mindfulness**: Being present in the moment rather than dwelling on worst-case scenarios helps keep fear in check.

Real-Life Examples of Overcoming Self-Doubt and Fear

- **Starting a New Job**: It is normal to doubt your skills in a new role. Overcoming that doubt involves focusing on the experience and training you bring, seeking help when needed, and celebrating small achievements at work.
- **Speaking Up in Meetings**: Many people fear being judged if their ideas are not "perfect." Learning to voice an idea anyway—knowing it can be refined—helps break the cycle of silence and helps you grow.
- **Pursuing a Passion**: You might always dream of writing a book, launching a business, or learning to play an instrument. Self-doubt might say, "It's too late," or, "I'm not talented enough." But each time you write a page, plan a business idea, or practice a chord, you prove self-doubt wrong.

The Importance of Supportive People

While inner work is crucial, having a community or even a single person who believes in you can help tremendously. Surround yourself with people who encourage your growth and respect your journey. Talk openly about your fears and doubts. Their support can remind you that you are not alone.

Setting Boundaries with Unsupportive Individuals

Sometimes, people around you might fuel your fear or doubt. They may mock your goals or constantly point out potential failures. In these cases, setting firm boundaries is essential. You might reduce your interactions or explain that you need encouragement rather than constant doubt. If they do not respect this, you have the right to protect your emotional health by spending less time with them.

Transforming Doubt into Determination

Self-doubt can actually be turned into a form of motivation if you learn to use it wisely. Think of doubt as a sign that you care about doing well. Instead of letting it paralyze you, let it prompt you to prepare better. For instance, if you doubt your ability to pass an exam, you can channel that worry into studying more effectively rather than giving up.

Embracing "Nerves" as Energy

Professional performers often say they still feel nervous before going on stage, but they learn to interpret that feeling as excitement rather than a sign of doom. This shift in interpretation can make a huge difference in how you handle fear. Instead of viewing fear as a barrier, see it as a signal that you are about to do something meaningful.

Making Fear a Partner in Growth

It might sound strange, but you can treat fear as a partner rather than an enemy. Fear points out the edges of your comfort zone. Where fear appears, there is an opportunity to learn something new. If you see it this way, fear becomes a guidepost: "Here is a place I can grow."

Small Steps, Big Impact

Even tiny actions can help you break the hold of self-doubt. If you are afraid to speak up in a large meeting, start by sharing a small idea in a smaller group. If you dream of writing but feel stuck, try penning a short paragraph each day. Over time, these small steps add up, and you develop a track record of facing fear rather than running from it.

When Professional Help is Needed

Sometimes fear and self-doubt can be deeply rooted, especially if they come from past trauma or long-term anxiety. In those situations, it may be wise to seek help from a therapist or counselor. They can provide tools and techniques to help you reshape your thought patterns. There is no shame in asking for help; in fact, it shows courage and self-awareness.

Maintaining Momentum Against Doubt and Fear

Once you start making progress—taking small risks, challenging negative assumptions—it is important to keep going. Doubt can creep back if you become too comfortable. Think of personal growth like riding a bike uphill. If you stop pedaling, you risk rolling backward. Continuing to face fears, even in small ways, keeps your resilience strong.

Celebrating Your Progress

Make sure to acknowledge how far you have come. It is easy to focus on what still scares you or what you have not achieved yet. But celebrating your successes, no matter how small, builds self-confidence. It also reminds you that you are capable of taking on challenges again in the future.

Conclusion: Stepping Beyond Fear

Overcoming self-doubt and fear is a journey that never really ends, but each step forward brings you greater freedom. By gathering evidence of your capabilities, challenging perfectionism, gradually facing your fears, and practicing self-compassion, you build a reservoir of inner strength. This strength allows you to see fear not as a dead end but as a stage in your ongoing growth.

When you recognize that doubt is just a thought—and fear is just an emotion—you become less tied to them. You can acknowledge their presence but continue to move toward your goals. In the next chapters, we will look at how setting healthy boundaries, learning self-compassion, and releasing perfectionism can further deepen your self-acceptance and confidence. Keep going. Each time you face your fear, you grow a little stronger.

CHAPTER 7: SETTING HEALTHY BOUNDARIES

Healthy boundaries are like invisible lines we draw around ourselves for emotional, mental, and sometimes physical protection. These boundaries help us maintain respect and well-being in relationships—whether at home, at work, or in our community. When you know how to set boundaries, you tell the world how you want to be treated. You also protect your time, energy, and self-worth. Without boundaries, life can become filled with stress, resentment, and confusion. In this chapter, we will talk about what boundaries are, why they matter, and how to set and maintain them.

What Are Boundaries?

Boundaries are rules or guidelines you create about how people can behave around you. They help define what is acceptable or unacceptable in your interactions. For example, you might have a boundary that you do not answer work emails after 8 p.m., or you might have a boundary about what topics you are comfortable discussing with certain family members. Boundaries are personal—what feels right for one person might feel too strict or too loose for someone else.

Different Kinds of Boundaries

1. **Physical Boundaries**: These are about your physical space and body. For instance, you might not want certain people to hug you or enter your room without knocking.
2. **Emotional Boundaries**: These involve your feelings. If someone often criticizes you or makes you feel guilty, you could set an emotional boundary by telling them you will not continue a conversation when it becomes hurtful.
3. **Time Boundaries**: You decide how you spend your time and who you spend it with. If a friend keeps calling late at night and it disrupts your sleep, you might tell them you can only chat before bedtime.

4. **Material Boundaries**: These deal with possessions—like your car, computer, or money. For example, you might decide you will not lend money to people unless you feel sure you can afford to lose it.

Why Boundaries Matter for Self-Acceptance

When you set a boundary, you communicate that your comfort and well-being are important. This act alone is a statement of self-respect. People with strong self-acceptance know that their time and emotional health deserve protection. On the other hand, if you never set boundaries, you might end up feeling used, drained, or angry. This can harm your self-esteem over time, making you question your worth. Boundaries help you honor yourself.

Signs of Weak Boundaries

- You often say "yes" to things you do not want to do, just to avoid conflict.
- You feel guilty when you cannot meet someone else's demands.
- You allow people to invade your personal space or disrespect your opinions without speaking up.
- You are not sure how to express discomfort or how to ask for what you need.

How to Identify Your Boundaries

Before you can set boundaries, you need to figure out what they are. This can be a surprising process because many of us do not think about boundaries until they are crossed.

1. **Notice Your Feelings**: Pay attention to moments when you feel uneasy, annoyed, or stressed in a relationship. That discomfort often signals a boundary issue.
2. **Ask "Why?"**: When you feel upset or resentful toward someone, ask yourself why. Maybe you feel they are not respecting your time or privacy. Understanding the core issue is key.
3. **Reflect on Your Values**: Boundaries often connect to core values, like respect, honesty, or independence. If your value is honesty, you might set a boundary about not tolerating lies or half-truths in close relationships.

Communicating Your Boundaries

Setting boundaries is not just in your mind; you usually need to communicate them. Telling someone about your boundary can feel scary, especially if you fear their reaction. But clear communication is necessary to maintain healthy relationships.

Be Direct and Brief

You do not have to over-explain or apologize for your boundary. A simple statement like, "I am not okay with discussing that topic" or "I cannot lend you money right now" is often enough. If the person asks why, you can decide whether you want to explain more. However, feeling obligated to justify your boundary in detail can make you look uncertain or invite arguments.

Use an Assertive Tone

Being assertive means respecting both yourself and the other person. You do not have to be rude or confrontational. Instead, you can speak calmly and firmly: "I need this from our conversation," or "I appreciate your interest, but I am not comfortable sharing more details right now."

Expect Some Pushback

People who are used to you having no boundaries might react negatively when you start setting them. They might complain, act offended, or try to make you feel guilty. This reaction is common because you are changing the "rules" they have known for a long time. Stay firm. Over time, they may learn to accept this new arrangement.

Examples of Boundary-Setting in Everyday Life

- **Workplace**: You might tell a colleague, "I can answer emails until 5 p.m., but after that, I focus on family time."
- **Friendships**: If a friend wants to vent about their problems for hours every day, you can gently say, "I care about you, but I have limited time tonight. Can we talk for 15 minutes and then I need some personal downtime?"

- **Family Gatherings**: Maybe you have an uncle who always asks personal questions you do not want to answer. You can politely respond, "I am not comfortable talking about that" and change the subject.

Handling Guilt When Setting Boundaries

Guilt often arises after you set a boundary, especially if the other person is upset or surprised. You might worry that you were too harsh or that you are hurting the relationship. But remember, healthy boundaries should not harm a genuine connection. In fact, they protect it from resentment. It is normal to feel a bit uneasy at first, but with practice, you will see that setting boundaries is an act of caring for yourself and others.

How to Ease Guilt

1. **Remind Yourself Why**: Focus on the reasons you set this boundary. Maybe you need more rest or you want to protect your emotional health.
2. **Practice Self-Compassion**: Acknowledge that growth can be uncomfortable, but that does not mean it is wrong.
3. **Check the Outcome**: Often, after setting a boundary, things improve. You might find you have more energy for genuine interactions. That can help reduce guilt over time.

Respecting Other People's Boundaries

Boundaries go both ways. Just as you want others to honor your limits, you should honor theirs. If someone says, "I need time alone," or "I do not want to talk about that," try to respect it. Not only does this show empathy, but it also builds trust. You become someone they know they can be real with.

Boundaries vs. Walls

There is a difference between healthy boundaries and building walls. Walls are rigid: they shut out everyone and everything, often out of fear of being hurt. Boundaries, on the other hand, are more flexible. They let good things in while keeping harmful behavior out. Setting a boundary does not mean you are closing yourself off from people; it means you are guiding how you connect.

Signs of a Wall

- You refuse to share any personal information or emotions with anyone, ever.
- You end relationships quickly at the first sign of conflict, without trying to talk it through.
- You keep people at a distance out of a constant fear of being hurt.

Walls might seem to protect you from pain, but they often lead to loneliness and missed chances for genuine connection. Boundaries strike a healthier balance.

Adjusting Boundaries Over Time

Your boundaries might change as you grow. At certain times, you may need stricter boundaries—like if you are healing from a tough experience and need more personal space. At other points, you might feel more open. It is okay to review your boundaries and adjust them if your life situation changes. This does not make you inconsistent; it makes you adaptable.

Common Challenges in Boundary-Setting

Fear of Conflict

Many people avoid setting boundaries because they do not want arguments or tension. But remember, short-term discomfort can prevent long-term problems like resentment or burnout. In a way, small conflicts now can stop bigger conflicts later.

People-Pleasing Habits

If you grew up believing you must always be kind, polite, or helpful, saying "no" might feel almost impossible. You might worry people will think you are selfish. But real kindness includes kindness to yourself. Overextending yourself can lead to mental exhaustion and hidden anger.

Not Knowing You Have the Right

Some folks do not realize they have the right to say no, to ask for respect, or to protect their time. They might have grown up in families where personal boundaries were not recognized. Learning that you have the right to choose how you want to be treated is a major step in self-acceptance.

Practical Steps to Strengthen Your Boundaries

1. **Start Small**: You do not have to tackle the most daunting boundary first. Maybe begin with something minor, like telling a coworker you cannot do them a favor when you are already overloaded.
2. **Prepare Scripts**: If you are worried about how to phrase your boundary, practice a short line beforehand. For example, "I'm sorry, but I can't stay late today" or "I would rather not discuss my finances."
3. **Keep It Simple**: Do not over-apologize or give a long explanation. State your boundary calmly. If pressed, repeat it.
4. **Enforce the Consequences**: If someone repeatedly crosses your boundary, decide on the consequence. This might mean leaving the conversation, blocking their number, or seeking help from HR at work. Consistency shows you are serious.

Learning to Say "No"

Saying "no" is one of the hardest boundaries for many people. We fear disappointment, or we think we are being rude. Yet a clear, respectful "no" can actually prevent bigger issues. If you say "yes" but cannot actually fulfill the commitment, you create stress for both you and the other person. Honesty is better, even if it causes brief discomfort.

Examples of Polite "No" Responses

- "Thanks for asking, but I can't make it this weekend."
- "I'm honored you thought of me, but I have too much on my plate right now."
- "I appreciate the offer, but that doesn't work for me."

Recognizing Signs of Unhealthy Relationships

Sometimes, no matter how well you set boundaries, certain people will continue to ignore them. This can be a sign of an unhealthy relationship. If someone constantly bullies, disrespects, or manipulates you, stronger measures may be needed. You might have to limit your interactions or, in extreme cases, end the relationship. This step is never easy, but protecting your well-being is crucial.

Boundaries in Digital Spaces

In today's world, a lot of our interactions happen online. Setting boundaries there is just as important. You might decide you do not want to share certain personal details on social media, or you set a limit on how many hours you spend browsing. If someone sends you messages that make you uncomfortable, it is within your rights to block them or ask them to stop.

How Boundaries Boost Self-Acceptance

When you set healthy boundaries and see people respecting them, you feel more confident in your worth. You realize that you do not have to sacrifice your comfort or values to be loved or accepted. Over time, this strengthens your sense of self. You become someone who values their own needs without apology.

A Simple Boundary Exercise

Try this short activity:

1. **Think of One Area** in your life where you often feel drained—maybe a friend who always wants favors or a co-worker who gives you tasks that are not your job.
2. **Identify the Boundary** you would like to set. Perhaps it is, "I am only willing to help with personal favors once a week," or "I will not reply to work messages after 7 p.m."
3. **Plan Your Words**: Write down exactly how you will communicate this boundary. Keep it brief and clear.
4. **Decide on Consequences** if the person does not respect it. For example, you might politely refuse any additional request or send a reminder

message: "I've mentioned I'm busy after 7 p.m., so I'll address this tomorrow."
5. **Put It into Action**: The next time the situation arises, follow through on your boundary. Notice how it feels to stand up for your needs.

Giving Yourself Permission

Sometimes, the biggest hurdle to setting boundaries is believing you have permission to do so. If you have gone through life putting everyone else's wishes ahead of yours, it might feel wrong to place limits. But remember, self-acceptance includes honoring your own limits. Remind yourself daily: "I have the right to set boundaries for my well-being."

When Boundaries Are Tested

People who want something from you—time, energy, money, or attention—may try to test or push past your boundary. They might make you feel selfish or uncaring. Stand firm. You do not have to be rude, but do not back down just because someone is unhappy. If your boundary is fair and well-thought-out, you have every right to keep it in place.

Balancing Boundaries and Flexibility

Setting boundaries does not mean you can never help others or compromise. Being flexible is fine if it does not harm your well-being. For example, you might decide that normally you do not work on weekends, but once in a while, for a special project, you make an exception. The difference is you choose this exception freely, not out of guilt or fear.

Conclusion: Embracing Boundaries as Self-Care

Boundaries are a form of self-care that helps you honor your worth. They protect your energy, time, and emotional health, allowing you to thrive. While it might feel uncomfortable at first—especially if you are used to saying "yes" to everything—practice and patience make boundary-setting easier. Over time, you will see that people respect you more when you respect yourself. Your relationships become healthier, and you gain a deeper sense of peace and confidence in who you are.

In the next chapter, we will explore the concept of self-compassion. While setting boundaries is one way to show care for yourself, learning self-compassion will help you treat yourself gently, especially when you face setbacks. Together, boundaries and compassion act like two pillars that support true self-acceptance.

CHAPTER 8: LEARNING SELF-COMPASSION

Self-compassion is the practice of being kind and understanding to yourself. It is about recognizing that mistakes, failures, and difficult feelings are a normal part of being human. Many of us are quick to offer support or comfort to a friend who is struggling, yet when we face the same challenges, we judge ourselves harshly. Self-compassion allows you to extend that same warmth to yourself instead of harsh criticism.

What is Self-Compassion?

Self-compassion involves three main elements:

1. **Kindness to Yourself**: Treat yourself like you would treat someone you love. When you stumble, you do not rush to name-calling or judgment. You step back, take a breath, and offer gentle words of understanding.
2. **Common Humanity**: We remember that everyone suffers. Everyone has problems, fails sometimes, and feels sadness. By seeing that we are not alone in our struggles, we become less likely to view ourselves as "broken."
3. **Mindfulness**: Mindfulness is the act of being present with your feelings without judging them. Instead of pushing away pain or getting lost in it, you acknowledge your emotions as they are.

When these three elements come together, you create a nurturing space inside yourself.

Why Self-Compassion Matters for Self-Acceptance

Without self-compassion, self-acceptance can feel superficial. You might say you accept yourself, but the moment you make a mistake, you dive back into self-blame. True self-acceptance means embracing the good, the bad, and the messy parts of who you are. Self-compassion is like a soft cushion that supports you when you fall, reminding you that you are still worthy of kindness, no matter what.

The Cost of Being Self-Critical

Harsh self-criticism might feel like it pushes you to do better, but it usually has the opposite effect. Constant blame or shame can lead to anxiety, depression, and even physical health problems. Moreover, it can stop you from taking healthy risks or trying new things because you fear the crushing voice that might appear if you fail.

Recognizing the Inner Critic

We have covered negative self-talk before, but self-compassion focuses on how we respond to that negativity. Do you let it run wild? Do you fight it back with anger? Or do you gently acknowledge it and move toward a kinder perspective?

Techniques to Manage the Inner Critic

- **Pause and Observe**: When a critical thought appears, take a mental step back. Notice what triggered it.
- **Label the Thought**: Sometimes saying, "Here is that critical voice again" can stop you from becoming overwhelmed.
- **Offer Compassion**: Speak to yourself as you would to a dear friend. "I hear you're upset and scared, and that's okay. Let's figure this out together."

Exercises to Cultivate Self-Compassion

1. The Self-Compassion Break

Whenever you feel stressed or frustrated with yourself, pause and ask:

1. "What am I feeling right now?" (Name the emotion: anger, sadness, disappointment.)
2. "Everyone feels this way sometimes." (This is the common humanity piece—knowing you are not alone.)
3. "What is the kindest response I can give myself?" (Perhaps, "It's okay to make mistakes. I can learn and do better next time.")

2. Writing a Letter to Yourself

Take a few minutes to write a letter to yourself about something you are struggling with. Imagine you are writing to a close friend who feels bad about this same issue. Use supportive, loving words. Acknowledge their pain and remind them they are more than their mistakes. Then read the letter back to yourself. Notice how it feels to receive that kindness.

3. Self-Soothing Actions

Sometimes words are not enough. You might need physical comfort, like placing your hand over your heart, giving yourself a gentle hug, or even wrapping yourself in a cozy blanket. Think about what simple gesture would help you feel calmer in moments of self-criticism or anxiety.

The Role of Mistakes in Self-Compassion

One of the biggest barriers to self-compassion is how we treat mistakes. We might see errors as proof that we are not good enough. But mistakes are an inevitable part of learning and growth. When you practice self-compassion, you start to view mistakes as teachers instead of confirmations of your flaws.

Turning Mistakes into Learning

Instead of asking, "Why am I so terrible at this?" you ask, "What can I learn from this?" That small change in language can make a big difference in how you feel and how you move forward. It keeps you focused on progress rather than shame.

Healing Old Wounds with Self-Compassion

Some people struggle with self-compassion because they carry old wounds from the past—maybe from a family member who was very critical or a situation where they felt deeply embarrassed. Self-compassion can act like a gentle balm on these old hurts. When those memories resurface, respond with kindness instead of reliving the shame.

A Simple Reflection

Think back to a painful memory. Picture yourself as you were then—maybe younger or less experienced. What would you say to that version of you now, knowing what you know about self-compassion? Write it down. Remind yourself that even then, you deserved understanding and empathy.

Common Myths About Self-Compassion

Myth 1: It Makes You Lazy or Weak

Some people fear that being too kind to themselves will result in complacency. They think that harsh self-talk keeps them motivated. Research suggests otherwise. People who practice self-compassion often show more motivation and better resilience because they do not waste energy on beating themselves up.

Myth 2: It's the Same as Self-Pity

Self-pity is dwelling on your problems and feeling alone in them. Self-compassion, however, involves recognizing that everyone struggles and that you can still extend kindness to yourself through those struggles. It is not about dwelling; it is about caring enough to seek growth and healing.

Myth 3: It's Selfish

Caring for yourself does not mean ignoring others. In fact, when you are kinder to yourself, you often have more emotional resources to be kind to others. You cannot pour from an empty cup.

Incorporating Self-Compassion Into Everyday Life

Morning Routine

Start your day with a simple affirmation: "I will treat myself with kindness today, no matter what happens." This sets the tone for a more compassionate mindset.

During Challenges

When something stressful happens at work or at home, pause for a moment. Take a deep breath. Remind yourself: "This is hard, but I can show myself understanding and respect." Then think of a small, supportive action you can take.

Before Bed

Reflect on the day without judgment. If you made mistakes, offer yourself compassion: "I didn't handle that conversation well, but I'm human, and I can try better next time." End the day with a note of kindness toward yourself.

Building Compassionate Self-Talk

Compassionate self-talk means shifting the way you speak internally. Instead of hurling insults at yourself, you choose words that reflect patience, love, and hope. For many people, this is not natural at first—it takes real effort. But like any skill, it becomes easier with practice.

Balancing Compassion and Accountability

Being compassionate does not mean you ignore the need to make amends or solve problems. If you hurt someone's feelings, for instance, self-compassion can help you face it honestly. You can say, "I made a mistake. I feel sorry about it. I will apologize and see how I can fix this." Compassion ensures you handle errors without punishing yourself.

Observing Personal Growth Through Self-Compassion

As you become more compassionate toward yourself, you might notice changes:

- **Lower Stress Levels**: You spend less time fretting over your shortcomings and more time finding solutions.
- **Better Relationships**: You become less defensive because you do not feel the need to protect yourself from constant judgment.
- **Increased Willingness to Learn**: Mistakes do not scare you as much, so you are more open to new challenges.

- **Balanced Emotions**: You allow yourself to feel sadness or disappointment without letting it define your worth.

Helping Others Through Self-Compassion

When you practice self-compassion, you model a healthier approach to struggles. If you have children, they see how you handle mistakes or stress without falling apart in guilt. If you have friends going through a tough time, you can genuinely encourage them to be kind to themselves because you know the value of that approach. In this way, your personal growth can ripple out to benefit those around you.

Breaking the Cycle of Shame

Shame is the feeling that there is something fundamentally wrong with you. It is different from guilt, which usually focuses on a specific action. Shame makes you believe you are worthless, and it can trap you in a negative cycle. Self-compassion breaks that cycle by telling you that yes, you might have flaws or regrets, but you remain worthy of love and kindness.

Recognizing Shame Triggers

Shame can arise in certain settings or around certain people. Maybe you feel ashamed when your boss criticizes your work or when a family member points out a habit. Notice these triggers and remind yourself that you are more than any one error or habit. You can acknowledge the problem while still holding onto the truth that you deserve respect.

Self-Compassion in Times of Change

Big changes—like moving to a new city, changing careers, or going through a breakup—can stir up feelings of doubt. You might question your decisions or your ability to cope. Self-compassion can be a steady anchor in these times of transition. When life shifts around you, you can still rely on the kindness you show yourself. This inner support helps you remain calm and open-minded while you navigate the unknown.

A Small Self-Compassion Ritual

Try this brief ritual each week:

1. **Pick a Quiet Spot**: Maybe your bedroom or a peaceful corner in your home.
2. **Light a Candle or Play Soft Music** (only if it helps you relax).
3. **Reflect on One Challenge** you faced recently. It could be a mistake, a moment of self-doubt, or a conflict.
4. **Speak Kind Words** to yourself as if you are comforting a dear friend. You might say, "I'm proud of you for trying," or "It's okay that it didn't go as planned."
5. **Take a Deep Breath**: Let yourself feel any emotions that come up. Remind yourself that you are worthy of compassion.

Doing this regularly can strengthen your self-compassion muscles.

The Ongoing Journey

Self-compassion is not a finish line you cross. It is an ongoing process of remembering to be kind to yourself, especially when life is hard. Some days, you will handle challenges with ease; other days, you might slip into old habits of self-criticism. That is normal. Each time you catch yourself being harsh, you have another chance to practice compassion.

Moving Forward with Compassion and Acceptance

As we near the end of this chapter, remember that self-compassion helps you see your own humanity clearly. You are allowed to stumble and learn. You are allowed to feel pain without denying your worth. This gentle attitude forms a strong basis for self-acceptance, letting you exist in a more peaceful, confident state of mind.

In the coming chapters, we will keep building on these ideas. We will explore letting go of perfectionism, healing from past hurt, and strengthening self-belief in a way that supports the compassion you are cultivating. Continue forward, knowing that every act of kindness you show yourself is a step toward lasting peace and confidence.

CHAPTER 9: LETTING GO OF PERFECTIONISM

Perfectionism is the belief that you must do everything perfectly—or at least appear perfect—to feel worthy. It is an exhausting mindset that can hurt your confidence and keep you from true self-acceptance. Many people do not even realize they are perfectionists. They may think they are simply "motivated" or "trying to do their best." While aiming high can be good, perfectionism crosses the line into harmful territory when mistakes become unacceptable, or when you tie your self-worth to unrealistically high standards.

In this chapter, we will explore what perfectionism is, how it can sneak into daily life, and why letting go of it is important for self-acceptance. We will also discuss practical ways to free yourself from its tight grip so that you can be kinder to yourself.

Recognizing the Signs of Perfectionism

Perfectionism can hide under the mask of being "hardworking" or "detail-oriented." There is nothing wrong with caring about details or trying to do things well. However, perfectionism often shows up with certain warning signals:

- You feel constant pressure to avoid mistakes at all costs.
- You struggle to celebrate your achievements because you focus on tiny flaws.
- You delay or avoid tasks because you fear not doing them flawlessly.
- You feel a deep sense of failure if something does not turn out exactly as planned.

These habits can drain your energy and cause ongoing stress. There is a difference between having high standards and obsessing over never messing up. One is healthy, allowing room for growth and learning; the other is rigid, leaving you feeling never good enough.

Why We Become Perfectionists

Perfectionism often starts from an early age. Maybe you received praise only when you performed well in school or sports. Or perhaps you faced criticism each time you made a mistake, so you learned that mistakes are unacceptable. Sometimes culture, media, or social groups push the idea that you should always appear flawless—whether in looks, achievements, or personality. Over time, these messages can harden into the belief that anything less than perfect is a failure.

Fear of Not Being Enough

At the heart of perfectionism is often a fear that you are not enough. You might think, "If I am not perfect, people will see my flaws and reject me," or "If this project has any mistakes, I will lose respect." This fear can drive you to overwork, overthink, or over-plan, all to escape the possibility of judgment or disapproval.

Control and Certainty

Perfectionism can also come from wanting total control. When life feels uncertain, some people try to manage that anxiety by making every detail perfect. Yet the world is not fully in our control—mistakes, accidents, or surprises can still happen. The more we try to control everything, the more anxious and frustrated we become when things go differently than planned.

The High Cost of Perfectionism

Emotional Exhaustion

Constantly aiming for perfection can wear you out. You might feel drained because you are never satisfied, or because you keep redoing tasks to get them just right. This exhaustion can lead to burnout, irritability, and even physical health problems over time.

Missed Opportunities for Growth

If you refuse to try something unless you can do it perfectly, you might never try new things at all. You stay in your comfort zone to avoid mistakes, missing the chance to learn. Perfectionists often end up stuck, because moving forward means risking failure, which feels unbearable.

Strained Relationships

Perfectionism can also harm your relationships with others. If you hold people to impossibly high standards, they may feel judged or inadequate around you. On the flip side, you might avoid close connections because you do not want anyone to see your imperfections. Over time, this can lead to loneliness or tense relationships.

Shifting Your Mindset: Progress Over Perfection

One of the biggest steps in letting go of perfectionism is learning to value progress over perfection. This mindset shift involves recognizing that growth happens through trial and error. You do not suddenly become skilled or successful without going through stages of messing up and learning.

When you focus on progress, mistakes become stepping stones rather than proof of failure. You still care about doing well, but you do not link your entire self-worth to the outcome. It takes practice to adopt this viewpoint, especially if you have held onto perfectionist beliefs for a long time. However, each time you find yourself obsessing over a flaw, you can pause and ask, "Am I growing here? What did I learn?"

Practical Strategies to Let Go of Perfectionism

1. Set Realistic Goals

Instead of aiming to do everything perfectly, try setting goals that focus on learning or improving. For instance, if you want to learn a new language, avoid saying, "I must speak with zero mistakes in three months." Instead, set a goal like, "I will practice 20 minutes a day, five days a week, and track my progress." This approach values effort and consistency over a flawless outcome.

2. Accept That Mistakes are Inevitable

It might help to write down a reminder: "I will make mistakes. That is part of being human." Place it where you can see it daily—on your mirror, fridge, or desk. Accepting the reality of mistakes does not mean you do not care; it means you understand mistakes happen in the journey of growth.

3. Prioritize Tasks

Perfectionists often try to do everything perfectly, leading to stress and overwhelm. Practice prioritizing. Ask yourself which tasks truly matter. If you spend an extra hour making a simple report look perfect, but it leaves you with no energy for important family time, you might be putting your energy in the wrong place. Learning to let some things go undone or done "good enough" frees up space for what truly matters.

4. Track Small Wins

Make a habit of noticing small achievements each day. If you completed a chapter of a book you are writing, made a healthy meal, or made one small improvement in your exercise routine, celebrate it. This trains your mind to look for progress rather than dwell on shortcomings.

5. Practice Self-Forgiveness

When you do make a mistake—or perform below your own standards—actively choose to forgive yourself. Talk to yourself kindly. For example, "I did my best with what I knew at the time. I can learn from this and do better next time." Self-forgiveness cuts perfectionism off at its roots, because you are no longer punishing yourself for imperfection.

Changing Your Inner Dialogue

We have already discussed creating a positive inner voice in earlier chapters. That same approach applies to combatting perfectionism. If you catch yourself thinking, "I'm a failure because I messed this up," replace it with, "I wish it had gone better, but this does not define me. I can adjust and try again." Over time, your mind will become more flexible, and you will find it easier to bounce back from errors.

Embracing "Good Enough" in Daily Life

Learning to say "this is good enough" can feel uncomfortable at first for a perfectionist. However, this phrase is not about settling for low standards—it is about recognizing when you have done your best for the moment or when further improvement will not significantly change the outcome. This skill can be particularly helpful in everyday tasks. For example, if you spend hours trying to make your presentation slides perfect, ask if they are already clear and understandable. If yes, it might be time to stop tweaking tiny details.

The Link Between Perfectionism and Anxiety

Perfectionism often goes hand in hand with anxiety. You worry about failing, being judged, or not living up to expectations. This anxiety can stop you from enjoying the present moment because your mind is focused on preventing future mistakes. By letting go of perfectionist demands, you reduce the pressure that causes constant worry. This can lead to a calmer, more peaceful approach to daily life.

Learning from Role Models Who Embrace Imperfection

Look for examples of people who openly share their mistakes or failures. Some of the world's most successful individuals—artists, entrepreneurs, athletes—talk about the times they messed up and how those moments helped them grow. Reminding yourself that even accomplished people fail can break the illusion that perfection is the norm. It also gives you real-life evidence that great things can arise from embracing imperfection.

Supporting Others in Overcoming Perfectionism

When you start releasing perfectionism, you can also encourage others to do the same. If a friend is beating themselves up over a small mistake, offer a gentle reminder that perfection is an impossible standard. Share stories of your own failures and how they helped you learn. Creating a more accepting environment lifts everyone up.

When Professional Help Might Be Needed

Sometimes perfectionism is so deeply rooted that it causes severe anxiety, depression, or eating disorders. If you find that your perfectionist thoughts are harming your health or relationships, it might be wise to speak with a counselor or therapist. They can offer personalized strategies and help you explore the deeper reasons behind your need for perfection. Reaching out for help is not a sign of weakness; it is a step toward healing.

Daily Reminders and Affirmations

Here are a few gentle statements you can tell yourself daily (feel free to adapt them to your situation):

- "I am allowed to learn through mistakes."
- "My worth is not measured by my achievements."
- "I choose growth over impossible standards."
- "I can do my best without demanding perfection."

Repeating these reminders helps you gradually shift your mindset.

Building Confidence Through Imperfection

You might worry that letting go of perfectionism will make you lazy or careless. Actually, when you stop fearing mistakes, you often become braver and more creative. Instead of holding back, you try new ideas. You work hard, but not out of fear—you do it out of genuine interest or passion. This shift tends to build real confidence over time, because you see that you are capable even if everything is not flawless.

Practicing Self-Compassion Alongside Letting Go

In the last chapter, we explored self-compassion. This practice ties closely to releasing perfectionism. Each time you catch yourself being overly strict or condemning yourself for a minor slip, invite compassion instead. Think: "I'm human. I did my best in this moment. I can learn from it, but I will not beat myself up." This mindset creates a supportive inner environment where you can safely try, fail, and grow.

Real-Life Example of Progress Over Perfection

Imagine you want to learn painting. A perfectionist mindset might say, "My first painting must look like a masterpiece." If it does not, you might feel you have no talent and give up. But if you embrace imperfection, you see your first painting as step one. Yes, it may look messy, but you can discover what brushstrokes work and which colors blend nicely. Over time, each painting improves. You allow yourself to enjoy the learning process rather than demanding instant brilliance.

Letting Go Day by Day

Overcoming perfectionism is not something you do all at once. It is a day-by-day shift in how you view challenges, mistakes, and your own value. Some days, you might slide back into old perfectionist habits. That is okay. Each time you catch yourself, remind yourself of your new perspective. With repetition and patience, this more accepting attitude becomes your natural way of being.

Conclusion: Finding Freedom in Imperfection

Learning to let go of perfectionism can feel like taking off a heavy backpack you did not realize you were carrying. Suddenly, you can breathe easier. You have more energy for what truly matters—genuine growth, creativity, and meaningful connections. Perfectionism might have made you believe you had to earn your worth through flawless performance. But in truth, you are already worthy, whether you achieve all your goals or not.

CHAPTER 10: HEALING FROM PAST HURT

Everyone has a past filled with moments of joy and moments of pain. Some painful experiences may fade with time, while others remain like open wounds. Healing from past hurt is a key part of self-acceptance because we cannot fully accept ourselves if we are stuck in old shame, anger, or sadness. In this chapter, we will explore ways to process and release emotional pain from the past, and how doing so can help you move forward with more confidence and peace.

Understanding Emotional Wounds

Emotional wounds can come from many sources: childhood trauma, betrayal by a friend, a painful breakup, or a harsh comment that cut you deeply. These hurts leave marks on our self-esteem and can shape our beliefs about ourselves and the world. For instance, if someone you loved abandoned you, you might develop a fear of abandonment in future relationships. If a parent repeatedly told you that you were not good enough, you might carry a sense of unworthiness into adulthood.

How Wounds Affect Our Present

1. **Recurring Negative Thoughts**: Unresolved pain can show up as negative beliefs about yourself—like "I am unlovable" or "I always fail."
2. **Overreaction to Triggers**: You may react strongly to certain words, places, or situations that remind you of your past hurt, even if the present situation is not harmful.
3. **Self-Sabotage**: Sometimes, old pain leads you to sabotage your own happiness. You might avoid close relationships or new opportunities because you fear repeating past hurts.

Choosing to Heal

Healing does not mean forgetting what happened or pretending it did not hurt. It means you decide to face the pain, acknowledge it, and work through it. This process can be challenging. You might feel strong emotions like anger, grief, or fear. But healing also brings relief, freedom, and a renewed sense of self.

Giving Yourself Permission

Many people resist healing because they feel they do not have the right to move on. They might think, "My pain is too big," or "It happened so long ago, I should be over it by now." But healing takes however long it takes. Giving yourself permission to heal is the first step. You deserve emotional freedom, regardless of how big or small the hurt seems to others.

Methods of Healing

1. Acknowledging the Hurt

Some people try to bury past pain. They distract themselves with work, entertainment, or other activities. While this can provide short-term relief, the hurt often resurfaces. Acknowledging your pain means admitting it is there. You might do this by writing about it, talking to a trusted friend, or even quietly reflecting on it during a walk. Recognizing that you are hurt is not weak; it is courageous because it allows you to start the healing process.

2. Expressing Emotions Safely

Unexpressed emotions can weigh you down. Finding a safe way to express them—like journaling, art, music, or speaking with a counselor—helps you release built-up tension. For example, writing a letter (which you do not need to send) to the person who hurt you can help you sort through your feelings. Or you might paint or draw how you feel, letting colors and shapes represent emotions that are hard to put into words.

3. Seeking Professional Help

If the pain is deep or connected to trauma, talking with a therapist can be a life-changing step. Therapists are trained to guide you through processing painful memories. They can offer coping strategies tailored to your situation, whether that involves cognitive-behavioral therapy, trauma-focused therapy, or another approach. Seeking help is not a sign of weakness. It shows you value your well-being enough to invest in professional support.

4. Practicing Mindfulness

Mindfulness involves staying present in the moment, without judging whatever thoughts or feelings arise. When painful memories pop up, instead of trying to push them away or drowning in them, you notice them with gentle curiosity. Ask yourself, "What am I feeling right now? Where is this feeling in my body?" By observing your emotions, you give them space to be felt and eventually released, rather than running from them.

5. Considering Forgiveness (If It Feels Right)

Forgiveness can be misunderstood. It does not mean you pretend the hurt never happened or that you excuse harmful behavior. Rather, forgiveness means choosing not to let the pain control your life anymore. It is about releasing the heavy emotional baggage so that you can move forward. This can involve forgiving someone who wronged you, or even forgiving yourself for mistakes you made in the past. It is a personal choice, and you should never feel forced to forgive if you are not ready. But for many, forgiveness is a powerful tool for healing.

Letting Go of Shame

Shame is a particularly sticky emotion. It tells you there is something fundamentally wrong with who you are. If past hurt made you feel unworthy or flawed, working through that shame is essential. One way is to remind yourself that you were in a situation where you likely did the best you could with what you knew at the time. You are allowed to have compassion for the person you were back then. That does not mean you approve of everything that happened—it means you recognize your humanity.

Dealing with Anger

Anger is a common emotion tied to past hurt. You might feel anger at the person who hurt you or anger at yourself for not seeing it coming. While anger can be valid and sometimes protective, holding onto it for a long time can poison your mental state. Finding healthy ways to process anger—such as talking with a counselor, writing about your feelings, or engaging in physical activity—helps you transform anger into a stepping stone for growth. It might even guide you to set stronger boundaries or advocate for yourself more confidently.

Honoring Your Healing Pace

Healing is not a straight line; it is more like a winding path with ups and downs. Some days you might feel great, ready to move on, and other days you might feel the old pain flare up unexpectedly. This is normal. It does not mean you are failing at healing. You are simply human, and emotional wounds can take time to fully mend. Try to be patient with yourself. Celebrate small steps, like going a week without feeling triggered or noticing that your reactions to reminders of the hurt are less intense.

Rewriting Your Story

Sometimes, we form a story around our hurt that defines who we are: "I am the person who was betrayed," or "I am the one who always gets abandoned." While acknowledging your experiences is important, it does not have to define your entire identity. You can rewrite your story to include growth, resilience, and new beginnings. For instance, you might say, "Yes, I was hurt, but I learned to stand up for myself and trust again."

Building a Supportive Environment

Just as we learned about setting boundaries in an earlier chapter, your healing journey can be supported or hindered by the people around you. Surround yourself with individuals who respect your process and avoid those who belittle your feelings or pressure you to "get over it" quickly. If you do not have supportive family or friends nearby, consider joining a support group (in-person or online). Hearing from others with similar experiences can be both comforting and empowering.

Reclaiming Trust

If your past hurt involved a betrayal, regaining trust in others can feel daunting. Start by trusting yourself—your instincts, your capacity to make decisions that protect your well-being. Over time, you can practice trusting small things in new relationships, like sharing a minor secret and seeing if the other person respects your privacy. As you see signs that some people are trustworthy, you can gradually open up more. This process can be slow, but each positive experience helps rebuild your belief in connection.

Healing the Inner Child

Sometimes, pain from childhood lingers into adulthood. If you had a difficult upbringing or faced abuse, a part of you might still feel stuck in those old fears. Healing your "inner child" can involve visualization—imagining yourself comforting and protecting the younger version of you. You might also use affirmations like, "I am safe now. My feelings matter. I deserve care." Over time, this gentle approach can soften the scars of childhood trauma.

Embracing Hope

Healing from past hurt does not mean you will never feel sadness about what happened. You may always carry a small ache for what was lost. But healing replaces the heavy weight of pain with a sense of hope and acceptance. You learn that you are not forever broken, and that new possibilities can arise even after deep hurt. This hope becomes a light guiding you toward a fuller, happier life.

Signs You Are Making Progress

- You find yourself thinking about the event or person less often.
- When memories do come, they feel less overwhelming.
- You can talk about what happened without feeling intense shame or anger.
- You catch yourself smiling or laughing more, enjoying the present.
- You feel more compassionate toward yourself and others.

Moving Forward With Self-Acceptance

Once you begin to heal, you may notice a shift in how you see yourself. Instead of viewing yourself as a victim or someone defined by hurt, you realize you are strong, capable, and deserving of peace. This new perspective allows deeper self-acceptance to take root. You do not deny the hardships you faced—you simply refuse to let them keep you from embracing your worth.

Combining Healing with Other Self-Acceptance Tools

Healing from past hurt is not separate from the rest of your self-acceptance journey. It works alongside setting boundaries, practicing self-compassion, and releasing perfectionism. Each of these tools supports the others. As you heal, you become more compassionate toward yourself. As you become more compassionate, it becomes easier to set boundaries and let go of perfectionism. The result is a stronger, more peaceful sense of self.

Allowing Joy After Pain

A final note: many people who have gone through deep hurt struggle to let themselves feel joy again. They might worry that if they become happy, something bad will happen to take it away. Or they may feel guilty about moving on, as if enjoying life dishonors the seriousness of their past. But embracing joy is an important part of healing. It shows that your hurt does not have the final say. You can carry the lessons from your past while still dancing, laughing, and loving freely in the present.

Conclusion: Turning Pain into Strength

Healing from past hurt can transform your life. Though it may involve tears, memories, or tough conversations, each step you take breaks another chain holding you back. You learn that you are resilient—that you can feel pain and still rise. As you leave behind the weight of old wounds, you open space in your heart for self-acceptance, hope, and new possibilities.

CHAPTER 11: STRENGTHENING SELF-BELIEF

Self-belief is the feeling inside that tells you, "I can handle what comes my way." It is different from pride or arrogance, which make you think you are better than others. True self-belief is about trusting that you have the ability to learn, adapt, and keep going even when things get hard. It is also about knowing that your worth does not crumble if you stumble or fail. Strengthening self-belief is essential for self-acceptance because it helps you see yourself as capable and resilient, rather than always doubting who you are.

In this chapter, we will explore ways to build self-belief in a sincere, lasting way. We will talk about how your thoughts, habits, and small daily actions can shape the trust you have in yourself.

Why Self-Belief Matters

Imagine driving a car on a long trip. If you do not believe the car can make the journey, you might never get on the road. That is how self-belief works in life. If you do not trust yourself, you might not try new things or push past challenges. You may remain stuck in the same routines or avoid growth because you fear you will fail. But when you believe in yourself, you open the door to possibilities. You feel you can try, learn from mistakes, and keep moving forward.

The Link to Self-Acceptance

If you do not believe in your own abilities, you may struggle to accept yourself fully. You might think, "Why should I accept someone who cannot achieve anything?" This negative thought could keep you from seeing your true worth. However, as you develop self-belief, you begin to see that you have strengths and talents. You also recognize that you can grow in areas where you are not strong yet. That balanced view leads to deeper acceptance of who you are.

Factors That Weaken Self-Belief

Doubt Passed Down

Sometimes, a lack of self-belief can come from words others said to you in the past. Maybe you had a teacher or relative who doubted your abilities, telling you, "You're not going to succeed," or "You can't do that." Hearing these statements at a young age can plant seeds of doubt that continue to grow over time.

Fear of Failure

We may also lose self-belief by fearing failure. If you think a single failure means you are not capable, you might avoid doing anything that risks failing. Over time, this avoidance can shrink your self-belief even more, because you never get to test your abilities in new areas.

Perfectionist Thinking

Earlier, we discussed letting go of perfectionism. Perfectionists sometimes tie their worth to perfect results, so if they achieve less than 100%, they feel useless. This mindset can weaken self-belief because small mistakes feel like big confirmations of not being good enough.

Shifting from Self-Doubt to Self-Belief

Recognize Your Achievements (Big and Small)

One helpful step is to make a note of what you have already accomplished in life. These accomplishments do not have to be huge. They could be times you solved a hard puzzle, helped a friend in need, learned a new skill, or tackled a personal challenge. Remind yourself that you did those things. This shows you have the ability to make things happen, even if you sometimes doubt yourself.

Set Yourself Up for Small Wins

If your self-belief is shaky, it can help to pick challenges that stretch you just a bit beyond your comfort zone. Maybe you decide to cook a new meal if you usually rely on takeout, or you volunteer to lead a small part of a project at work.

These challenges are small enough to feel achievable but big enough to give you a sense of growth. Each time you succeed at a new, modest challenge, your self-belief grows.

Practice Balanced Thinking

Balanced thinking means noticing both what you do well and what you can still improve. It is neither overly positive nor overly negative. If you succeed at something, allow yourself to feel proud rather than brushing it off. If you fail, do not label yourself as incapable; instead, treat it as a learning opportunity. This balanced view stops your mind from jumping to extremes like "I am the best" or "I am worthless."

Building Supportive Mental Habits

Positive Self-Talk

Negative self-talk can crush self-belief. If you constantly call yourself names or say, "I can't handle this," your mind begins to believe it. Changing that to more encouraging words can make a huge difference. For instance, if you catch yourself saying, "I'll never learn this," pause and switch to, "I'm just starting, and I can figure it out step by step."

Imagining Success

Visualization can also help strengthen self-belief. Take a moment to imagine yourself successfully completing a task you are nervous about. How do you feel during and after finishing it? How do you deal with obstacles? By practicing this mental exercise, you give your brain a preview of success. This can ease anxiety and boost belief in your ability to carry things through.

Being Kind to Yourself

Self-compassion is a close friend of self-belief. When you offer yourself kindness, you send a message that you are worth caring for, even when you struggle. This softens the fear of failure and encourages you to keep trying new things. If you slip up, you do not berate yourself; you simply recognize you are learning and deserve understanding.

Action Steps for Strengthening Self-Belief

1. Keep a Progress Journal

Write down moments where you felt proud, did something well, or pushed through a challenge. You can look back on these notes when doubt creeps in. Over time, you will build a record of your wins—proof that you can rise to various situations.

2. Celebrate Effort, Not Just Results

It is easy to tie all your confidence to outcomes. But if you focus only on results, you miss all the steps you took along the way. Celebrating effort means you feel good about trying your best, regardless of the outcome. This can be especially helpful if you are doing something brand new and not yet skilled at it.

3. Seek Support When Needed

Sometimes self-belief can grow when you talk with encouraging friends, mentors, or even a professional counselor. They can point out strengths you may overlook and remind you of times you conquered challenges. They can also help you develop realistic goals and stay accountable to your progress.

4. Face Your Fears Gradually

If there is a specific fear holding back your self-belief—like fear of public speaking, fear of learning a new software, or fear of social rejection—you can practice facing it step by step. Start with the easiest scenario, then build up as your confidence grows. Each step you accomplish confirms your capability, chipping away at doubt.

Overcoming Obstacles to Self-Belief

Dealing with Criticism

Not everyone will believe in you. Some people might criticize or mock your efforts, whether out of their own insecurities or simple negativity. While it can sting, it is key to remember that their words do not define you. Constructive criticism can be helpful if it shows you how to improve. But general insults or mean comments often reflect more about the person speaking them than about you.

Coping with Setbacks

Even with a strong sense of self-belief, setbacks happen. Maybe you get rejected from a job or lose at a competition. These moments can shake your confidence. To handle them, remind yourself that a single loss does not erase your strengths or your future possibilities. If needed, take a short break to regroup, then return with a fresh perspective and a plan to move forward.

Balancing Self-Belief with Humility

Strengthening self-belief does not mean you become arrogant or ignore feedback. Arrogance usually involves thinking you are always right and better than others. Healthy self-belief is about trusting your abilities while staying open to learning from mistakes or from more experienced people. This balance makes it easier to connect with others and continue growing.

Self-Belief in Different Areas of Life

Work and Career

When you trust yourself at work, you may volunteer for new projects or share ideas in meetings without second-guessing your every word. This can lead to growth in your career, as people notice your willingness to learn and contribute.

Personal Goals

Self-belief helps with personal goals like fitness, learning an instrument, or traveling to new places. You do not quit at the first sign of difficulty. Instead, you push on, knowing you can overcome obstacles or at least learn a lesson in the process.

Relationships

Having faith in yourself can also improve friendships and romantic relationships. If you believe in your own worth, you are less likely to stay in unhealthy relationships or let others treat you poorly. You respect yourself, which sets a standard for how you expect to be treated.

A Personal Exercise: The Mirror Talk

Try standing in front of a mirror, looking into your own eyes, and stating aloud something you believe you are good at or a quality you admire in yourself. It might feel strange at first, but hearing your own voice speak positively can reinforce your sense of worth. For instance, you could say, "I am learning more every day, and I'm proud of how I handle new challenges." Over time, this exercise can become a supportive habit.

Common Myths About Building Self-Belief

Myth: You Either Have It or You Do Not

Some people think self-belief is an inborn trait—you are either born confident or insecure. That is not true. Self-belief grows with practice, life experiences, and a conscious decision to challenge negative thoughts.

Myth: A Single Success Will Fix Everything

While a big success can boost your confidence, real self-belief is built on multiple experiences. One achievement does not create a permanent shield against doubt. Instead, consistency in trying, learning, and seeing progress shapes long-term self-trust.

Myth: Self-Belief Means Ignoring Weaknesses

Having faith in your abilities does not mean ignoring areas where you need work. In fact, people with strong self-belief are usually more willing to face their weaknesses, because they trust they can improve. They see weaknesses as opportunities, not reasons to give up.

Checking In with Yourself

Sometimes, it helps to do a quick mental check about your current level of self-belief. Ask yourself questions like: "Am I avoiding something because I feel I can't do it?" or "Have I discredited my progress by focusing only on mistakes?" If you find that doubt is creeping in, take a moment to recall your past wins or remind yourself of the skills you do have. This small step can stop a downward spiral of negative thinking.

Spreading Belief to Others

When you grow in self-belief, you can also help others believe in themselves. You might encourage a friend who feels uncertain about a new job or hobby. You can share your own journey, explaining how you fought self-doubt. This creates a positive cycle: as you lift others up, you also reinforce your own confidence.

Self-Belief as an Ongoing Journey

Like many things in life, building self-belief is not a one-time event. You do not just "get confident" and stay that way forever. You will face new challenges and sometimes doubt yourself again. That is normal. Each time you overcome a challenge, you add another layer of trust in yourself. Over years, you build a strong foundation that can weather bigger storms. So, do not be discouraged by bumps along the way.

Putting It All Together

Strengthening self-belief is about treating yourself as someone who can learn, adapt, and achieve. It involves noticing your achievements, celebrating your efforts, and facing your fears step by step. Even if you fail at times or hear criticism, self-belief reminds you that your worth is not tied to one outcome. You can always grow, improve, and find new paths.

As you apply these ideas to your life, you may discover hidden strengths. You might try activities you once avoided, speak up more at work, or explore deeper connections in your relationships. Self-belief acts like a gentle hand guiding you from inside, reminding you that you are not stuck, you are capable, and you have every right to trust your journey.

With this stronger sense of self, we can now turn to the next chapter, which focuses on practicing mindfulness for inner peace. Strengthening your self-belief makes it easier to remain calm and focused in the present moment, and mindfulness further boosts your self-acceptance by teaching you to accept what is happening without harsh judgment. Together, these skills create a powerful support system for real peace and confidence in your everyday life.

CHAPTER 12: PRACTICING MINDFULNESS FOR INNER PEACE

Mindfulness is a way of paying attention to what is happening right now, without judging it. When you practice mindfulness, you step away from worries about the future or regrets about the past. Instead, you calmly notice your thoughts, feelings, and surroundings as they are. This gentle awareness can bring a sense of inner peace that helps you accept yourself more deeply. By letting go of mental clutter and focusing on the present, you create room for clarity and ease.

In this chapter, we will explore what mindfulness looks like in day-to-day life, why it is useful for self-acceptance, and how you can start or deepen your own mindfulness practice.

Understanding the Core of Mindfulness

At its core, mindfulness is about being fully present. That might sound simple, but many people spend much of their time lost in thought—planning their next move, reliving old failures, or worrying about what others think. Mindfulness invites you to notice these thoughts and then gently bring your focus back to the here and now.

Common Misunderstanding

Some people think mindfulness means "emptying your mind" or "never thinking." That is not accurate. The mind naturally thinks. It is its job, just like the heart's job is to beat. Mindfulness involves noticing thoughts without getting sucked into them. You do not try to force them away; you simply observe them, then let them pass, returning your focus to the present moment.

Why Mindfulness Helps with Self-Acceptance

Breaking the Cycle of Negative Thoughts

When you are mindful, you notice negative thoughts—like "I'm not good enough" or "I always mess up"—as they pop up. But instead of believing these thoughts, you see them as passing mental events. This perspective gives you a chance to question their truth or redirect your focus, rather than getting trapped in a spiral of negativity.

Building Compassion Toward Yourself

Mindfulness can also include paying attention to your emotional states. If you are feeling upset, you simply notice, "I'm feeling sadness" without judging yourself for it. This nonjudgmental attitude often leads to greater self-compassion. You realize it is okay to have emotions; it does not make you flawed. This gentle acceptance of your feelings translates into a deeper acceptance of yourself.

Reducing Stress and Anxiety

A lot of stress comes from imagining worst-case scenarios or reliving past mistakes. By staying present, you reduce the power these imagined problems have over your mind. You learn that in the "now," you are usually safe and capable of handling what is actually happening. Over time, this lowers anxiety, allowing you to be calmer and more open.

Simple Ways to Practice Mindfulness

1. Mindful Breathing

One of the easiest ways to start is by focusing on your breath. You can do this almost anywhere—while sitting at your desk, riding a bus, or lying in bed. Take a moment to feel the air move in and out of your nostrils, or notice how your belly rises and falls with each inhale and exhale. If your mind wanders, gently bring it back to the breath without scolding yourself.

2. Body Scan

A body scan involves mentally scanning your body from head to toe, noticing sensations. Do you feel tension in your shoulders? A slight ache in your back? Warmth in your hands? You observe these sensations without trying to fix them right away. This practice makes you more aware of how your body holds stress or comfort and can help you release tension.

3. Mindful Eating

Instead of rushing through meals, try eating mindfully. Take smaller bites and chew slowly, noticing the taste, texture, and smell of your food. Pay attention to how your body feels as you swallow and wait for your next bite. This simple act can transform routine meals into a calming, pleasant experience, and it also helps you listen to your body's signals about hunger and fullness.

4. Walking Meditation

If you prefer movement, walking meditation might suit you. Choose a quiet place, walk slowly, and pay attention to how your feet touch the ground with each step. Notice your surroundings—like the rustle of leaves or the breeze on your skin—without labeling them as good or bad. Each step becomes a moment of awareness.

Integrating Mindfulness into Everyday Life

Mindfulness is not only for formal practice like meditation sessions. You can bring it into daily tasks: washing dishes, brushing your teeth, or folding clothes. The key is to focus on what you are doing, using your senses to stay present. If your mind drifts, gently bring your attention back. This helps you find calm moments in the busiest of days.

Using Reminders

One practical tip is to set up small reminders. For example, place a sticky note on your bathroom mirror that says "Be here now," or set an hourly reminder on your phone to pause for a few mindful breaths. These nudges help you remember to return to the present moment before stress or negativity can pile up.

Overcoming Common Hurdles

Restlessness

When you first try mindfulness, you might feel restless. Sitting still and focusing on your breath can be tough if you are used to constant activity. This restlessness is normal. Instead of fighting it, notice it: "I feel restless." Then gently return to your focus. Over time, the restlessness often decreases.

Doubts and Expectations

Sometimes people expect that mindfulness will instantly solve all their problems or make them feel eternally blissful. While mindfulness can bring noticeable benefits, it is not a magic fix. It is a skill that develops gradually. If you find yourself doubting whether it "works," observe that doubt in a mindful way and continue practicing anyway.

Frustration with Wandering Thoughts

Your mind will wander—guaranteed. You might plan dinner, remember a conversation, or worry about tomorrow's meeting, all during a mindfulness session. This does not mean you have failed. Each time you notice your mind has wandered and bring it back, you are practicing mindfulness correctly. Think of it like training a puppy to come back when called. You are building a mental muscle.

How Mindfulness Supports Inner Peace

Slowing Down Reactive Habits

When you are not mindful, you might react to stress in automatic ways—maybe snapping at someone or reaching for junk food. Mindfulness creates a small gap between trigger and response. You become aware of your emotion before you act on it. This gap gives you a chance to choose a healthier response, building more peaceful relationships and habits.

Accepting Yourself in the Present

A big part of mindfulness is acceptance—accepting what you see, feel, or think in the current moment. Over time, this acceptance expands beyond the moment to include accepting yourself. You stop fighting who you are or what you feel, and instead, you learn to work with it gently. This mindset shift can heal self-criticism and foster genuine peace with who you are.

Deepening Your Practice

Guided Meditations

If you find it hard to practice on your own, try guided meditations. Many apps, websites, or online videos offer step-by-step guidance, letting you follow along as a calm voice walks you through breathing, relaxation, or visualization. This support can help you stay focused until you get more comfortable.

Mindful Journaling

Writing can also be a form of mindfulness. Pick a few minutes each day to write down what you are feeling or noticing in the present. Keep your tone nonjudgmental, as if you are an observer of your own thoughts and emotions. This method can help you sort through complicated feelings without getting stuck in them.

Attending Mindfulness Workshops or Retreats

If you want a more immersive experience, consider a mindfulness workshop or a retreat. Spending a day or weekend in a structured environment with an experienced teacher can deepen your understanding and give you a stronger foundation. These events often include group practice, talks, and personal reflection time.

Connection to Other Self-Acceptance Skills

Mindfulness works hand in hand with the topics we have explored in earlier chapters:

- **Self-Compassion**: Mindfulness helps you notice when you are being harsh with yourself so you can replace that harshness with kindness.
- **Setting Boundaries**: When you are mindful, you are clearer on how certain interactions make you feel, which supports healthier boundary-setting.
- **Healing Past Hurt**: Mindfulness grounds you in the present, reducing the power past pain holds over you.

By combining mindfulness with these other skills, you form a strong base for well-being.

Finding Moments of Peace in Everyday Life

Pausing Between Tasks

Instead of rushing from one chore to the next, pause for 10 seconds in between. Take one slow breath, noticing how your body feels. This mini-break can refresh your mind and prevent feelings of overwhelm.

Mindful Listening

When talking with someone, really listen to their words instead of planning your response in your head. Notice their tone, facial expressions, and the feelings behind their words. You will likely understand them better and feel more connected. This also helps you stay present in conversations rather than drifting off.

Ending the Day Calmly

Before going to sleep, try a brief mindful activity. You could do a short body scan in bed, guiding your attention from your toes to your head. If a worrying thought about tomorrow appears, acknowledge it and gently bring your focus back to your breathing. This habit can improve sleep and help you end the day on a peaceful note.

How Mindfulness Boosts Confidence

When you are mindful, you are not comparing yourself to an ideal image in your head or someone else's social media feed. You are simply experiencing life as it is. You realize that many of the stories you tell yourself—like "I must be perfect to be loved"—are just thoughts, not facts. Seeing through these limiting thoughts frees you to be your genuine self. As a result, you grow more confident because you no longer measure your worth by unrealistic standards.

Mindfulness in Challenging Times

Life includes tough moments—arguments, disappointments, or personal crises. Mindfulness does not remove these obstacles. Instead, it teaches you how to face them without being swallowed by panic or anger. By taking a slow breath and anchoring in the present, you give yourself space to respond wisely rather than react impulsively.

Real-Life Example

Imagine you receive harsh feedback at work. Your normal response might be panic or anger, and you might fire back a defensive email. With mindfulness, you notice your heart rate speeding up and your face becoming hot. Rather than hitting "reply" right away, you take a few mindful breaths and observe your emotions. Once they settle, you might write a more constructive response or even wait until you are calmer to speak with your manager. This approach can preserve relationships and your own peace of mind.

Staying Motivated on the Mindfulness Path

It can be challenging to keep practicing mindfulness long-term, especially if life gets busy. One strategy is to remember why you started in the first place. Maybe you wanted to feel less stressed, be kinder to yourself, or live with more joy. Write down your reasons and read them occasionally to remind yourself of the benefits. You could also pair mindfulness with something you already do daily, like making your morning coffee. While waiting for it to brew, take a minute of mindful breathing.

Beyond the Individual: Mindful Communities

Some people like to join mindfulness groups or attend local meditation centers. Practicing with others can enhance motivation and provide a sense of community. You see that you are not alone in facing a busy mind or in seeking peace. Group discussions can also open your eyes to different ways people use mindfulness to handle difficulties.

Embracing the Ongoing Nature of Mindfulness

Like self-belief, mindfulness is a skill you build over time. You cannot perfect it in a day or a week. There will be times you feel very present and times your mind is all over the place. That is normal. Each time you gently bring your attention back to now, you strengthen your ability to live mindfully. You are growing—step by step, breath by breath.

Conclusion: Finding Ease Through Awareness

Practicing mindfulness opens a door to inner peace. You discover that much of your stress and unhappiness stem from dwelling on the past or worrying about the future. By focusing on what is happening right now—with acceptance and without harsh judgment—you give yourself a chance to feel calm, clear, and more at home with who you are.

This calm, accepting state reinforces all the work you have done to build self-acceptance, self-belief, and healthier relationships with others. It becomes easier to accept your flaws, celebrate your growth, and handle life's ups and downs. In the next chapters, we will look at finding your unique strengths, handling stress, and more practical steps that continue to deepen your self-acceptance journey.

Remember, mindfulness is not about being perfect at paying attention; it is about showing up to the present moment with openness. Each small moment of awareness adds up, leading to a healthier, more confident sense of self.

CHAPTER 13: FINDING YOUR UNIQUE STRENGTHS

We often hear people say, "Focus on your strengths." But if someone asks, "What are your unique strengths?" many of us freeze. We might think, "I do not have any special gifts," or "I am just average." The truth is, each person has a unique blend of talents, interests, and qualities that make them strong in ways they may not recognize at first. Finding these strengths is a powerful part of self-acceptance because it helps you see the parts of yourself that shine.

It is not always about being the best at something. Sometimes your strength shows up in how you handle tough times, in how you care for others, or in how you solve problems in creative ways. When you discover these abilities, you gain confidence and start trusting yourself more. The world feels more open because you see you have something valuable to offer, both to yourself and to those around you.

Why Finding Strengths Matters

Finding your strengths matters because it changes the way you see yourself. Instead of always focusing on flaws or things you think you cannot do, you turn your attention toward what you can do well. For a lot of people, this simple shift in focus can be life-changing. Maybe you grew up in a place where people mostly pointed out your mistakes. Or maybe you have been surrounded by peers who seemed more talented or successful, leaving you feeling overshadowed. By identifying your own strong points, you finally stop comparing yourself to others and start seeing your own path.

Focusing on strengths also fuels motivation. When you work with what you are naturally good at or interested in, you find more energy to keep going. Imagine pushing a heavy cart uphill versus rolling it on a flat road. The second situation flows more easily because you are not constantly fighting against an uphill climb. Your strengths are that flat road—using them keeps you from struggling against your own nature.

Overcoming the Fear of Seeming Boastful

One reason people struggle to see or share their strengths is the worry about seeming arrogant. They think that if they name their gifts out loud, they are bragging. But recognizing your strengths is not the same as bragging. Bragging is when someone tries to show off or make themselves seem better than everyone else. Simply saying, "I have a talent for writing," or "I am good at listening," does not put others down or make you superior. It is just an honest statement about what you do well.

In fact, identifying your strengths can be humble because you are also likely to notice where those strengths are needed. You may look at the community around you and think, "I am pretty organized, so maybe I can help plan an event," or "I am good at comforting people, so maybe I can volunteer at a support center." Using your strengths in service to others is anything but bragging—it is generosity in action.

Different Kinds of Strengths

When people think of strengths, they sometimes imagine skills like playing sports or singing. But strengths can show up in all sorts of ways. You might be skilled at creating art or fixing machines. You might have a knack for remembering details, or you might be great at talking to strangers. You could have a strong sense of empathy, making you good at understanding how others feel. Sometimes people do not see empathy, patience, or kindness as "strengths" because these qualities are not rewarded with trophies. Yet they are often the hidden gems that make a big difference in everyday life.

Some strengths are about personality—like being calm under pressure or being quick to laugh. Others are about learned abilities—like speaking multiple languages or knowing how to code. Still others are about character—like honesty, integrity, or determination. Take time to reflect on the wide range of possible strengths. This opens your eyes to gifts you might have overlooked.

Steps to Discover Your Strengths

Reflect on Past Successes

One simple step is to look back at times you felt proud of something you did. It could be a project at school or work, a personal goal you reached, or a kindness you showed someone. Ask yourself what qualities helped you succeed. Did you use creativity, patience, or bravery? Did you show leadership, or did you quietly support someone in need? These reflections hint at recurring patterns of strength.

Notice Moments of "Flow"

Sometimes you get so absorbed in an activity that time seems to fly by. This state, often called "flow," can be a clue about your strengths. Think about tasks where you lose track of the clock because you are deeply focused and enjoying yourself. Perhaps it is baking, writing, teaching, or solving puzzles. Flow suggests not only that you like doing something but also that you have natural abilities suited for it.

Listen to Compliments

People around you may sometimes notice your strengths more easily than you do. If family members, friends, or coworkers keep saying you are great at explaining things, or that you have a calming presence, take these compliments seriously. We often brush them aside out of modesty or disbelief. But these observations can shine a light on real talents you might be taking for granted.

Keep an Open Mind

Try to avoid ruling out strengths just because you think they are "not a big deal." The fact that something feels easy for you could be a sign it is indeed a strength. Maybe you find it simple to make people laugh or to organize messy spaces. What feels easy to you might be very hard for someone else, which indicates it is a special strength for you. Remember, not all strengths have to be flashy.

Strengths and Self-Acceptance

When you embrace your strengths, you begin to see that you bring something unique to the table. This recognition can quiet that little voice that says, "I am not good enough." Of course, you still have areas to improve—it is not about believing you are perfect. It is about seeing the whole picture of who you are, which includes not only flaws or past mistakes but also gifts and abilities worth celebrating.

Noticing your strengths can also help you set more honest goals. If you decide to use your knack for organization to start a new system at work, you set yourself up for success instead of frustration. If you enjoy comforting friends, you might lean into roles that let you use that gift more often, like volunteering at a helpline or studying counseling. That sense of alignment—between your strengths and your activities—often leads to a more satisfying life.

Handling Self-Doubt When Looking for Strengths

It is normal to feel doubt when you try to name your strengths. You might think, "But I am not really great at anything," or, "Maybe people just say I am good at this to be nice." Self-doubt can be a big hurdle. If you find it hard to trust your own evaluation, consider talking with a mentor, teacher, or friend who knows you well. Ask them what they see as your positive qualities or skills. Sometimes an outside perspective helps break through your own disbelief.

You can also practice writing down one small strength each day. Maybe you note, "I was patient with my younger sibling today," or "I managed a stressful meeting without losing my cool." Over time, these small notes become proof that you do have areas of strength, even if they do not sound spectacular. Remember, strength is not measured only in grand achievements; sometimes the best strengths show up in quiet daily behaviors.

Balancing Strengths and Weaknesses

Accepting your strengths does not mean pretending you have no weaknesses. Real self-acceptance involves seeing both sides. The good news is that playing to your strengths can often help you manage your weaker areas. For instance, if you are not good at detailed planning but you are strong at seeing the big picture, you might team up with someone who loves planning details. If you are shy in group settings but strong at one-on-one conversation, you might focus on smaller gatherings to share your ideas. Recognizing your strengths helps you find ways around or through your weaker spots.

At the same time, being aware of weaknesses is not a reason to feel bad about yourself. Everyone has them. The key is choosing which weaknesses you want to work on improving and which ones you will accept or work around. You cannot be great at everything, and that is perfectly okay.

Discovering New Strengths Over Time

Strengths are not frozen in place. As you grow older or explore new experiences, you might uncover strengths you did not know you had. Perhaps you discover a hidden love for storytelling after you volunteer to read books to children. Or maybe you find you have a real talent for leadership when you step up to organize a community project. Life events can draw out abilities that were lying dormant, waiting for a chance to shine.

This is one reason it is good to try new activities, even if you are not sure you will like them. Each new experience offers a chance to learn about yourself. Sometimes, you will realize, "No, this is not my strength," and that is also valuable information. Other times, you will be pleasantly surprised to find a skill that lights you up. Keeping an open mind allows your strengths to keep evolving.

Putting Strengths into Action

Once you know a few of your strengths, how do you use them? Start with your everyday life. If you are good at calming people down, you might make a habit of checking in with stressed friends or family members. If you are great with numbers, you might offer to help your neighborhood group with budgeting. If you have a creative side, maybe you volunteer to design posters for a local event. Using your strengths in day-to-day tasks builds your sense of identity and helps you practice self-acceptance through contribution.

Sometimes, using your strengths also opens doors professionally. Employers value unique skill sets, especially if you can clearly show how your abilities help the team or the company. Even if you are not in your dream job right now, weaving your strengths into your role can make your day more fulfilling and help you stand out in a positive way.

Avoiding Comparison

One trap people fall into after identifying strengths is comparing them to others. You might realize you are a pretty good singer, then immediately think of a friend who has an even more powerful voice. Or you might see your skill in cooking and then recall a famous chef on TV who is far beyond your level. This comparison can kill the joy of discovering your own abilities. Remember, your journey is yours alone. Being good at something does not have to mean you are the best in the entire world. Your strength still holds value, whether or not it is number one on some universal scale.

Focusing on personal growth instead of comparison also keeps your self-acceptance secure. You are not trying to measure up to a list of external standards. You are simply recognizing that you have qualities worth celebrating and that you can continue to grow in your own way. This mindset frees you from chasing impossible ideals and lets you take pride in exactly where you are.

Strengths in Relationships

When you know your strengths, you can also bring more honesty and balance to relationships. You are less likely to pretend to be someone you are not, because you know what you genuinely bring to the table. For instance, if you are a good listener, you can be the person friends go to for advice or just a kind ear. If you are more of a practical helper, you might offer to run errands for someone who is overwhelmed. Recognizing each other's strengths in a friendship or partnership can also avoid misunderstandings. Instead of expecting your partner to excel in something they do not enjoy, you appreciate the strengths they actually have, and they do the same for you.

A Quick Reflection Exercise

If you have paper or a journal handy, you can try a brief exercise to uncover strengths you might have missed:

Close your eyes, take a breath, and think of a moment from the past few weeks when you felt especially satisfied or happy with yourself. It does not need to be dramatic—it could be a tiny instance. Maybe you made someone smile or completed a small project on time. Write down exactly what happened. Then write what qualities you used in that moment. Did you show patience, humor, diligence, creativity, or calmness?

Doing this often can create a record of your lesser-known strengths. The more you do it, the more patterns you will see. You might realize you are consistently patient in tense situations or that you often use humor to ease awkwardness. Identifying these patterns is a big step toward embracing who you are.

Strengthening Self-Acceptance Through Awareness

You do not have to prove your strengths to anyone in order to accept them. Even if people around you do not notice or praise you for certain abilities, they can still exist and thrive. Self-acceptance grows when you validate your own positive qualities without waiting for external approval. You can think, "I have a warm, supportive nature, and that is enough for me to appreciate it, even if I do not get constant compliments."

When you stop looking for others to confirm your worth, you become more grounded in yourself. That sense of inner security is what allows real peace to flourish, because you are no longer anxious about who is noticing or not noticing your gifts. You have a quiet confidence that is not easily shaken by outside opinions.

Looking Ahead

In the broader journey of self-acceptance, knowing your strengths is a key piece of the puzzle. It balances out the self-awareness of your weaknesses or flaws. It boosts your motivation to chase goals that align with who you truly are. And it brings joy, because you begin to see life as a field where you can use your unique gifts rather than a place to hide your supposed shortcomings.

As you move forward, keep exploring your strengths in new ways. Dare to step into activities that excite you, even if they feel a bit outside your comfort zone. Often, our greatest strengths show themselves when we face new challenges. Embrace the fact that you are a work in progress. Your strengths are part of your story, helping you grow, connect with others, and find fulfillment in the day-to-day.

In the next chapter, we will dive into practical ways to deal with stress and anxiety. Recognizing and using your strengths can help reduce stress, but there are many other techniques and habits that also play a big role in creating inner calm. By combining your unique gifts with effective stress management, you strengthen the foundation of peace and confidence in your life.

CHAPTER 14: DEALING WITH STRESS AND ANXIETY

Stress and anxiety are common parts of life. Everyone feels them at some point, whether it is before an important test, during a major life transition, or when facing big responsibilities. While some degree of stress can motivate you to act, too much stress or ongoing anxiety can harm your mental and physical health. It can make you doubt yourself, lose focus, and feel tense all the time. In this chapter, we will explore ways to recognize and handle stress and anxiety in a healthy manner, so you do not let them overwhelm your sense of peace and self-acceptance.

Understanding Stress and Anxiety

Stress usually appears when you feel you have too many demands and not enough resources—time, energy, or knowledge—to meet them. Anxiety is a form of fear or worry about what might happen in the future, often coupled with physical reactions like a racing heart or tense muscles. Both stress and anxiety can serve as signals that something in your life needs attention. If you are worried about passing a test, it might be a sign to study more or manage your time better. But when they become constant or too intense, they can rob you of sleep, happiness, and the belief in your own ability to cope.

One key to self-acceptance is learning that feeling stress or anxiety does not mean you are weak. Emotions like these are normal. They are alarm bells telling you to pay attention. The challenge is to handle them in a balanced way, rather than letting them take over.

Why Stress and Anxiety Hurt Self-Acceptance

When stress or anxiety hits, you might blame yourself for feeling overwhelmed. You might think, "I should be stronger," or "Other people handle more than this, so why can't I?" This inner criticism can eat away at your self-confidence, making you feel as if you are failing at life. But remember, everyone has a limit to how much stress they can handle comfortably. Reaching that limit is not a sign of weakness—it is a sign that you are human and that your mind and body need support.

At times, anxiety also convinces you to avoid challenges because you fear failing. This avoidance can stop you from discovering new strengths or enjoying meaningful experiences. Over time, you might shrink your world to avoid discomfort, which can feed a sense of isolation or self-doubt. Dealing with stress and anxiety in a healthy way frees you to keep growing and exploring life.

Recognizing the Signs

Paying attention to your body and mind can help you notice when stress or anxiety is building up. Some common signs include tense shoulders, frequent headaches, trouble sleeping, irritability, or constant worry about small things. Maybe you find yourself snapping at loved ones for no real reason, or you spend hours replaying conversations in your head. These signals are your body's way of saying, "I am overloaded."

It helps to pause and identify triggers. Are you stressed because of an upcoming deadline? Are you anxious about social events? By spotting triggers, you can plan how to face them. Remember, awareness is the first step to managing any problem.

Healthy Ways to Manage Stress and Anxiety

Acknowledging Feelings

One of the most crucial steps is to admit that you are feeling stressed or anxious. Saying, "Yes, I am worried about this situation," is an act of honesty that starts the healing process. Pretending you are fine when you are not only pushes the stress deeper, allowing it to build in your subconscious.

Setting Realistic Expectations

Stress often comes from expecting too much of yourself in too little time. If you overload your schedule with tasks or set standards that are impossible to meet, you are inviting stress to run your life. Try to set goals and timelines that are challenging yet realistic. If you see you are hitting a wall, it might be time to reduce commitments or ask for help instead of pushing yourself to the edge.

Creating Breaks

The human body and mind need breaks to recharge. Working nonstop or filling every minute with tasks can lead to burnout. Whether it is a short walk, a quick stretch, or a moment to breathe quietly, these pauses can lower stress hormone levels and renew your energy. Building in small rests throughout the day might sound simple, but it can make a big difference in how you feel by evening.

Physical Activity

Activities like walking, dancing, or even a quick set of jumping jacks can help your body burn off tension. Exercise releases endorphins—chemicals in your brain that boost mood. This does not have to be intense. A gentle yoga session or a peaceful bike ride can work wonders. The point is to get your body moving, allowing physical energy to shift and calm your mind.

Supportive Connections

Talking to someone you trust about your worries can lift part of the burden. Whether it is a friend, family member, or therapist, sharing your thoughts out loud sometimes helps you see them in a clearer light. The listener might offer fresh perspectives or simply provide comfort by understanding your feelings. Human connection often reduces the feeling of being alone in your struggles.

Mindfulness Techniques

Earlier, we discussed mindfulness as a way to stay present. This skill is especially useful for dealing with anxiety, which loves to drag you into future "what if" scenarios. By focusing on your breath or senses in the current moment, you interrupt the loop of worrying thoughts. Even a minute or two of mindful breathing can create a calm pause in the middle of a stressful day.

Balanced Thinking

Anxiety sometimes runs wild with worst-case scenarios: "I will fail this test and never get a good job." Balanced thinking means asking yourself, "Is that really true, or is it just my fear talking?" It also means looking at possible positive outcomes or neutral outcomes. By reminding yourself that many outcomes are possible, you weaken the grip of anxiety on your mind.

Dealing with High-Pressure Situations

Sometimes stress is tied to big events—like a job interview, a performance, or a major exam. Preparing ahead of time can lower some of the tension. If you have an interview, practice your answers and do research on the company. If it is a performance, rehearse until you feel steady. For tests, plan a study schedule instead of cramming the night before. This practical approach gives you a sense of control, reducing the anxiety that arises from the unknown.

On the day of the event, let yourself feel a bit of adrenaline—that is normal. Adrenaline can help you focus. But also remind yourself that one event does not define your worth. If things do not go perfectly, it is not a final judgment on your abilities. That understanding alone can lift a lot of the pressure.

Handling Ongoing Anxiety

Some people experience ongoing anxiety that does not tie to a single event. They might feel a constant sense of worry or dread, even when there is no clear reason. This can be tied to generalized anxiety disorder or other conditions that benefit from professional help. If you find that anxiety or panic attacks are interfering with your daily life, talking to a mental health professional can be a wise step. Therapies, support groups, or even medication (if recommended by a doctor) can provide relief and coping strategies.

Seeking help is not a failure. It is a form of strength. Just as you would see a doctor if you had constant headaches or a broken bone, you deserve support for ongoing anxiety. Professional guidance can open doors to new methods of handling stress, from structured therapy approaches to lifestyle tips tailored to your situation.

Connecting Stress Management with Self-Acceptance

When you take steps to handle stress and anxiety, you show yourself that your well-being matters. This action alone boosts self-esteem, because it is a form of self-care. You are saying, "I am important enough to help myself feel better." Over time, this consistent care builds a foundation of respect for who you are, flaws and all. You recognize that you do not have to be stress-free all the time to be worthy—you simply need to respond to challenges with kindness and effort.

Moreover, by handling stress in healthier ways, you keep that negativity from feeding into thoughts of "I am a failure." You start to see stress or anxiety as events to manage rather than proof of your inadequacy. This shift in perspective can lighten your emotional load, making self-acceptance more natural.

Avoiding Unhealthy Coping

When stress or anxiety feels overwhelming, it is tempting to reach for quick fixes like overeating, drinking alcohol, or escaping into endless gaming. While these might numb the worry in the moment, they do not solve the root issue and can create new problems. Unhealthy coping can also hurt your self-view, as you might feel regret or guilt afterward.

Replacing these habits with healthier ones is crucial. For example, if you notice yourself wanting to binge on junk food when stressed, you could try a short walk or a craft activity instead. If you find yourself reaching for alcohol, you might choose to call a friend or dive into a relaxing hobby. The more you practice healthier responses, the more natural they become.

Dealing with Stress at Work or School

Work and school are common sources of stress. You might have deadlines, grades, or performance reviews on your mind. One approach is to break tasks into smaller steps. If you have a big project, list each part of it: research, outlining, drafting, revising. Tackle them one by one, celebrating each small finish. This helps prevent the sense of being swallowed by a huge, vague responsibility.

Another strategy is to communicate. If the demands on you are truly unrealistic, talking to a teacher, supervisor, or advisor might lead to a more reasonable workload. Sometimes people in charge do not realize how much they are asking until someone speaks up. Asking for an extension or clarifying expectations can ease some of the weight on your shoulders.

Social Anxiety and Self-Acceptance

Some stress comes specifically from social situations—like meeting new people, speaking in public, or attending gatherings. If social anxiety is a big challenge, it helps to practice in low-stakes environments. Maybe you start by having short, friendly chats with a coworker or by joining a small group activity rather than a huge party. Each positive experience builds confidence and teaches your brain that social interaction is not as scary as it seems.

Even if you do feel nervous in social settings, remind yourself that it is okay to take breaks. Step outside or find a quiet corner for a moment if you need to calm your nerves. You are not obligated to be "on" all the time. Recognizing your comfort level is part of self-acceptance, and others often respect that more than we fear.

Harnessing Relaxation Tools

Learning a few relaxation exercises can provide instant relief when anxiety spikes. Deep breathing—slowly inhaling, holding for a beat, then exhaling—sends a message to your body that it is safe to relax. Progressive muscle relaxation, where you tense and then relax different muscle groups, helps release physical tension. Visualizing a peaceful scene can also shift your mind away from stressful thoughts. These simple techniques can be done quickly, even in public places, without drawing attention to yourself.

Turning Stress into Growth

While stress and anxiety are uncomfortable, they can also be teachers. Sometimes, examining the cause of your stress reveals something that needs changing. Maybe your job is not a good fit, or a certain friendship is draining you. Or perhaps your schedule has no free time, leaving you on the edge. By listening to what stress is telling you, you might find clues to make healthier choices or realign your priorities.

Likewise, pushing through anxiety to try new things can lead you to discover strengths and experiences you might have missed otherwise. Each time you handle stress or cope with anxiety in a healthy way, you prove to yourself that you can adapt. This self-trust grows into deeper self-belief over time, reinforcing the lessons from previous chapters.

When to Seek Additional Help

Not all stress can be managed by personal efforts alone, especially if you are dealing with chronic anxiety or a life crisis. If you feel hopeless, unable to sleep for long periods, or as if your anxious thoughts never stop, consider reaching out to a mental health professional. Therapists, counselors, and psychiatrists are trained to help you navigate these deep waters. They can give you specialized strategies, whether through talk therapy, structured behavioral therapies, or medication if needed.

Seeking help is a strong step, not a sign of weakness. It shows you value your mental health and are willing to take action to protect it. Many people find that a combination of therapy and personal mindfulness or relaxation practices leads to long-term relief and a renewed sense of self.

Conclusion: Building Resilience for Calm and Confidence

Dealing with stress and anxiety is a process, not a one-time fix. Life will always throw new challenges your way, but each tool you learn—mindful breathing, balanced thinking, exercise, or seeking support—becomes a block in your resilience foundation. Over time, you will notice that while stress and anxiety still appear, they no longer shake your entire sense of self.

You start to see yourself as someone who can bend without breaking, someone who can feel scared yet move forward anyway. This view ties back into self-acceptance, because you realize it is okay to be imperfect and to have tough feelings. You are still worthy, still growing, and still able to find peace and confidence no matter what.

CHAPTER 15: BUILDING SUPPORTIVE RELATIONSHIPS

One of the most fulfilling parts of life is having a network of people who care about you—friends, family, and even colleagues who encourage you to be your best self. These are supportive relationships, and they can offer warmth, understanding, and respect. When you have supportive relationships, it is easier to accept yourself because you feel safe to be who you really are. In this chapter, we will explore ways to build strong connections with others, handle conflicts in a healthy manner, and ensure those relationships grow in a balanced way.

Understanding What Makes a Relationship Supportive

A supportive relationship is one in which both people feel comfortable expressing themselves honestly. This comfort might involve sharing joys, fears, and even mistakes without being judged. Such relationships often include the following traits:

1. **Respect**: Each person respects the other's boundaries, feelings, and opinions.
2. **Empathy**: There is a willingness to listen and try to understand what the other person is going through.
3. **Mutual Benefit**: Both individuals give and receive support, though not always in the exact same way or at the same time.
4. **Trust**: You can count on the other person to keep their word or keep your personal matters private.

When these qualities are present, you feel a sense of safety that allows you to be yourself. You do not have to pretend or hide your flaws. Instead, you can grow and learn within the relationship, knowing that you have someone in your corner.

The Importance of Genuine Connection

A genuine connection goes beyond formal introductions or superficial chats about the weather. It means you allow each other to see the real you. Genuine connection does not need to be dramatic or deeply personal right away. It can start with small, honest interactions—like admitting you have had a rough day or sharing a story about something that made you laugh. Over time, these moments of honesty add up, creating a bond that is stronger than small talk.

Recognizing Superficial Connections

Not every relationship will be supportive or genuine. You may have acquaintances with whom you only discuss surface topics. That is okay—these more casual connections can still serve a purpose in your social life. But it is important to recognize that you will not get the same level of support or personal growth from these connections as you would from a more genuine bond. Learning to tell which relationships have deeper potential allows you to spend more energy on those that uplift you.

Starting New Friendships and Bonds

Some people worry about making new friends or think that building a supportive network is too hard. However, remember that many others are also looking for genuine connection. If you remain open-minded and take small steps, you can find people who share your interests and values.

Finding Shared Interests

A great way to meet supportive individuals is by doing activities that you naturally enjoy. If you like painting, take a class or go to a casual art meetup. If you enjoy a certain sport, join a local club. By engaging in something that interests you, you are more likely to come across people with similar passions. Starting conversations becomes easier because you already share a topic you both care about.

Being Approachable

Approachability can make a difference when forming new bonds. This does not mean you have to plaster a fake smile on your face all the time. It simply means being open in your body language—uncrossing your arms, making gentle eye contact, and greeting others. A calm, friendly demeanor invites people to talk to you. Even a small act like asking if you can sit next to someone at a workshop or offering a passing greeting can open the door for conversation.

Nurturing Existing Relationships

Even if you already have friends or a partner, those relationships need ongoing care. Much like plants need water and sunlight to grow, relationships need time, respect, and thoughtful attention to stay strong. Here are ways to nurture them:

Regular Communication

Frequent contact does not have to be lengthy or deep every time. A quick text to say, "How are you doing?" can remind your friend or family member that you care. For closer relationships, you might plan calls or get-togethers so you can share updates about your lives. Consistency helps people feel valued. It also prevents misunderstandings or drifting apart over time.

Active Listening

Active listening is a powerful skill in relationships. When the other person speaks, try focusing fully on their words. That means not playing with your phone or letting your mind wander. Show that you hear them by asking follow-up questions or summarizing what they said. This makes the speaker feel understood and respected, which strengthens your bond.

Sharing Emotions and Thoughts

Supportive relationships flourish when both sides share not just facts but also feelings. It can be tempting to keep your worries or sadness to yourself, thinking you do not want to burden others. But letting close friends or family in on how you truly feel allows them to support you. In turn, they might open up about their own struggles. This mutual openness creates deeper trust.

Setting Boundaries Within Relationships

Earlier, we talked about boundaries. In supportive relationships, healthy boundaries are crucial. Even the most caring person needs a certain amount of privacy and independence. For instance, you might enjoy your friend's company but still need alone time. Communicating your boundaries clearly helps the other person understand your needs without guessing or feeling rejected. Boundaries also protect your sense of self, ensuring you do not lose your identity by merging too much with another person's preferences.

Recognizing Toxic or Unsupportive Relationships

Sometimes, a relationship can become harmful rather than supportive. Signs of a toxic relationship might include:

- Constant criticism or belittling.
- Control or manipulation—one person always insists on having things their way.
- Lack of respect for your boundaries, time, or emotions.
- Feeling unsafe or anxious when you are around the person.

If you notice these patterns, it is important to address them or even consider walking away from that relationship if it does not improve. Holding onto toxic relationships can damage your self-esteem and make it harder to accept yourself. You deserve connections that uplift, not drain, you.

Conflict and Healthy Resolution

No matter how close two people are, conflicts will happen. Maybe you disagree on how to spend time together, or one of you feels hurt by something the other said. Having a conflict does not mean the relationship is doomed. In fact, working through disagreements can make the bond stronger if done respectfully.

Tips for Handling Conflict

1. **Stay Calm**: Anger or raised voices often cause people to stop listening. If emotions run high, take a short break to breathe.

2. **Speak from Your Perspective**: Use "I" statements rather than "You did this!" For example, "I felt hurt when you forgot our plan" is more constructive than "You never care about my feelings."
3. **Focus on Solutions**: After expressing feelings, try finding a way forward together. Ask, "How can we prevent this problem next time?" or "What can we agree on?"
4. **Know When to Pause**: If the conflict feels too big or emotions are overwhelming, agree to revisit the topic later. Sometimes a bit of space can help each person gather thoughts and calm down.

Giving and Receiving Support

Support is not always about fixing someone else's problem. Often, it is about being present and acknowledging what the other person is going through. This can mean listening, offering a shoulder to cry on, or suggesting a new perspective when they are open to hearing it. At the same time, do not forget that you also need support sometimes. A supportive relationship goes both ways, but it is okay to lean on the other person when you need help. Let them be there for you; it is a gift they can give you, just as you give to them.

Growing Together Through Shared Activities

Spending quality time together can deepen supportive relationships. Consider doing something new as a team—like a cooking class, a weekend trip, or a small volunteer project. Shared experiences create fresh memories and give you both something to talk about. They also help you see different sides of each other. You might discover a friend's great sense of humor in an unexpected situation or notice how calm they are when faced with a challenge.

Balancing Relationships With Alone Time

Even when you love the people in your life, you still need space to connect with yourself. Alone time is not selfish. It recharges your energy, helps you reflect, and prevents burnout from constantly being around others. By maintaining a healthy balance of social interaction and solitude, you can show up more fully in your relationships. You are less likely to become irritable or feel smothered, and your friends or family will likely appreciate the healthier dynamic.

Handling Changes in Relationships

Over time, relationships evolve. Some friendships grow closer, while others drift apart. Sometimes people move to different cities, start families, or change life paths. These shifts can be bittersweet, but they are a natural part of life. Accepting that not every relationship will stay the same can save you from unnecessary worry or self-blame. If a once-close friendship fades because your interests diverge, it does not mean you or the other person did anything wrong—it might simply reflect a change in life circumstances.

Staying Connected From Afar

Even if physical distance grows, technology offers ways to keep in touch—through messages, calls, or video chats. If you want to maintain a bond, these tools can help you remain part of each other's lives. However, it requires effort from both sides. Agree on times to chat and treat those moments as important appointments, showing that you care enough to make it work despite the distance.

The Role of Family in Supportive Relationships

Family ties can be strong sources of support, but they can also be complicated. Sometimes family members naturally provide encouragement and love. Other times, family dynamics involve disagreements or past tensions that make closeness challenging. If you have a supportive family, appreciate that bond and be willing to share your appreciation with them. If your family relationships are less nurturing, setting boundaries might help you keep the peace while preserving your mental well-being. Remember, you can still find family-like support among friends or mentors if your relatives cannot meet that need.

Supporting Others Without Losing Yourself

If you are someone who loves to help, you might find yourself constantly giving advice or emotional support to friends, coworkers, or family members. While this is generous, be careful not to burn out. You cannot pour from an empty cup. Make sure you are taking care of your own needs so you can be present for others without sacrificing your emotional health. Sometimes that means saying,

"I understand you are upset, but I need some time to rest before we talk," or suggesting that they seek professional help if the issue is beyond your ability to assist.

Building Community

Beyond one-on-one relationships, a sense of community can boost your overall well-being. This might be a local group that meets for sports, a religious or spiritual community, or an online forum where members share common goals. Communities give you a broader circle of support, and they can expose you to new perspectives or events. Feeling like you belong to a larger group can soothe the loneliness that sometimes creeps in, even when you have a few close friends.

Apologizing and Forgiving

No relationship is perfect. Sometimes you might hurt someone's feelings or say something you regret. Apologizing sincerely can mend the bond. This means acknowledging what you did, expressing genuine remorse, and asking how you can make it right. On the flip side, if someone apologizes to you and is earnest, consider offering forgiveness. Holding onto grudges can poison a relationship and your own heart, making it hard to move forward. Forgiving does not always mean forgetting or excusing the behavior, but it does allow you to release the heavy weight of resentment.

Celebrating the Good Times

A supportive relationship is not only about helping each other through struggles. It is also about celebrating each other's achievements and joys. Cheer for your friend who lands a new job or your sibling who finishes a tough project. Send a thoughtful note or plan a small celebration. These moments of happiness strengthen your bond because you share in each other's positive life changes, not just the challenges.

How Supportive Relationships Enhance Self-Acceptance

When you are surrounded by people who see the best in you, it becomes easier to see those good qualities in yourself. If you have a friend who admires your sense of humor, you start to acknowledge that humor is part of who you are. Over time, the acceptance you receive from supportive relationships can encourage you to be kinder to yourself. You feel less need to hide your flaws or feel shame about them. Instead, you view them as normal parts of being human—just like your strengths.

At the same time, building supportive relationships does not mean you need outside approval to feel good about yourself. Rather, these relationships work alongside your own self-care efforts. They remind you that you are not alone and that your presence matters. When you stumble, they offer a hand. When you succeed, they clap for you. Such an environment makes the journey to self-acceptance smoother and more fulfilling.

Moving Forward

Building and maintaining supportive relationships takes patience and effort, but the rewards are huge. You create a circle of people who celebrate your growth, stand by you in storms, and appreciate you for who you are. These relationships act like a mirror—reflecting back the positive aspects of you that you might overlook on your own. In turn, you become a supportive mirror for them, reminding them of their own worth and potential.

As we continue our journey, the next chapter will address the concept of developing emotional resilience. Resilience is the ability to bounce back from difficulties, and relationships can play a big part in that process. When tough times come, having supportive people to lean on can greatly boost your resilience. Combined with the personal skills you will learn, it creates a strong fortress against life's storms, letting you stand firm in your self-acceptance, no matter what challenges arise.

CHAPTER 16: DEVELOPING EMOTIONAL RESILIENCE

Life does not always follow our plans. There are challenges, disappointments, and unexpected twists. Emotional resilience is what helps you keep going in the face of these obstacles. It is the ability to recover from difficulties, adapt to change, and regain a sense of balance when emotions run high. You do not have to be born with resilience; it can be developed over time. In this chapter, we will discuss what emotional resilience is, why it is linked to self-acceptance, and how you can strengthen this inner capacity step by step.

What Is Emotional Resilience?

Emotional resilience means you bounce back from stressful events instead of staying stuck in fear, anger, or sadness. Picture a rubber ball that bounces back each time it hits the ground, versus an egg that breaks upon impact. The resilient person is like that ball—they might feel the impact of a stressful event, but they do not shatter; they find ways to cope, heal, and continue forward.

Myths About Resilience

Some people think resilience means never crying or never feeling hurt. That is not accurate. Resilience does not remove your emotions or make you cold. It simply helps you handle them better. A resilient person can acknowledge pain, grieve, or get angry, but they do not stay in that emotional state forever. They process the feelings, learn what they can, and then move on.

Why Emotional Resilience Matters

When you develop resilience, you free yourself from being held hostage by life's ups and downs. Sure, you will still face tough times, but those experiences do not define your worth. You begin to see that a failure, loss, or mistake is something that happened, not who you are. This view is crucial for self-acceptance because it stops you from linking negative events to your self-esteem. Instead, you recognize that you are allowed to face hardship without believing you are a failure as a person.

Resilience also makes you braver. If you trust in your ability to handle difficulties, you are more likely to take healthy risks—like trying a new career path, moving to a new city, or speaking up for yourself. You know that even if things do not go perfectly, you have the inner tools to cope.

Elements That Build Resilience

Self-Awareness

One core element of resilience is knowing yourself. That includes understanding your emotional triggers and typical reactions. If you know that sudden changes at work spike your anxiety, you can prepare strategies for those moments—like breathing exercises or a quick chat with a supportive coworker. Self-awareness stops stress from catching you off guard.

Mindset of Growth

A person with a growth mindset believes they can learn and evolve through effort, rather than feeling their abilities are fixed. This mindset helps in tough times because you see hardships as learning experiences rather than permanent roadblocks. You might think, "I did not handle that well this time, but I can do better next time," instead of "I will never be able to handle this."

Adaptability

Adaptability means being flexible with your plans. Life can throw curveballs—a sudden illness, a job layoff, or an unexpected family issue. Adaptable people shift their approach, looking for a new path rather than clinging to what used to work. This flexibility keeps stress from piling up when old strategies fail.

Steps to Strengthen Emotional Resilience

1. Build Your Coping Toolbox

A coping toolbox is a set of methods you can use when stress hits. This might include:

- **Calming Techniques**: Deep breathing, gentle stretching, or listening to soothing music.
- **Distraction Activities**: Watching a funny show, coloring a simple design, or reading a lighthearted book to give your mind a break.
- **Physical Outlets**: Taking a walk, doing mild exercise, or even cleaning to release pent-up energy.

Keep this toolbox in mind or write it down so you remember you have options when you feel overwhelmed.

2. Practice Stress Inoculation

Stress inoculation is a method where you gradually face small, controlled amounts of stress to build up your tolerance. For example, if you have social anxiety, you might start by saying hello to a stranger at the store. Over time, you push yourself a bit more—joining a small social gathering, then a larger event. Each successful experience rewires your brain to believe, "I handled that; maybe I can handle more."

3. Set Realistic Goals

A small success can build your confidence, while an impossible goal can lead to self-defeat. By choosing goals that stretch you slightly but remain within reach, you create repeated experiences of accomplishment. Each success, even if minor, tells your mind that you are capable. This is resilience in action—knowing you can tackle challenges bit by bit.

4. Learn from Past Failures

Think of a past failure that once felt devastating. How did you move on from it? What did you learn in the process? Reflecting on how you overcame past setbacks shows you that you have done it before. This memory can serve as proof: if you overcame that obstacle, there is a good chance you can overcome the next one. Viewing failures as lessons rather than lifelong labels is a hallmark of resilience.

Emotional Resilience and Self-Care

If you are running on empty—no rest, poor nutrition, or no social support—it is harder to bounce back from life's knocks. Self-care is not a luxury; it is part of maintaining the physical and emotional energy that keeps you steady. A good night's sleep, a balanced meal, and regular breaks can make the difference between handling stress well and falling apart.

Even just a few minutes a day of quiet reflection—whether through journaling, meditating, or a quick walk in nature—can help you reset your mind. This short pause gives you space to process emotions before they overflow.

Seeking Help When Needed

Resilience does not mean doing everything alone. Sometimes the best way to bounce back is to lean on the strength of others. That might involve talking with a friend or family member, joining a support group, or reaching out to a counselor. If you face a crisis that feels too big to handle, seeking professional help is a wise and responsible move. Needing support does not make you weak—it shows you care enough about yourself to get the resources needed for recovery.

Handling Emotional Overload

There are moments when life piles on too much at once—a breakup, a job loss, an illness, and family conflict all happening in a short time. Even people who are normally resilient can feel overwhelmed. When this happens:

1. **Acknowledge the Overload**: Denying how big the problem is will only cause more stress.
2. **Break It Down**: Identify each issue separately. Sometimes sorting out the chaos in your mind helps you address one problem at a time.
3. **Look for Immediate Supports**: Are there friends, family, or community resources that can temporarily lessen some of the burdens?
4. **Be Kind to Yourself**: Recognize that this is a tough period. Avoid judging yourself for not functioning at your normal capacity.

Emotional Regulation Techniques

Emotional resilience hinges on how well you can regulate strong emotions like anger, anxiety, or sadness. This does not mean ignoring them; instead, it means finding healthy ways to express and reduce them. Some methods include:

- **Writing in a Journal**: Putting your feelings into words can bring clarity and ease emotional tension.
- **Artistic Expression**: Painting, drawing, or playing music can let you pour out emotions you cannot quite say.
- **Talking It Out**: Sharing your frustration or sadness with a caring listener can lighten the load.

When you have a regular outlet for emotions, they are less likely to build up until they explode or cause numbness.

The Role of Mindfulness in Resilience

Mindfulness, as discussed before, helps you observe your emotions without being swallowed by them. When a stressor arises, you can pause, notice your racing heart or swirling thoughts, and simply name them: "I am feeling anxious." This small step creates space between you and your emotional storm. From there, you can choose a response rather than reacting blindly. Mindful awareness keeps you from exaggerating your troubles, allowing you to face them with more calmness.

Turning Pain into Purpose

Sometimes, resilience involves finding meaning in hardship. This does not mean you enjoy or seek out suffering, but rather that you notice how struggles can lead to personal growth. Maybe you learn humility, patience, or empathy through a tough experience. Or you find that going through pain inspires you to help others in similar situations. By turning pain into purpose, you transform a negative event into something that enriches your character.

Stories of Resilience

It can be helpful to think of people you admire who have overcome difficulties—whether a family member, a historical figure, or a community leader. These stories remind you that humans are capable of bouncing back from illness, poverty, heartbreak, or countless other challenges. You do not have to be famous to be resilient; everyday people show resilience in small, personal ways, like getting up each morning after a heavy loss or working hard to build a stable future after facing setbacks.

You might even reflect on your own life stories. Identify a time you were knocked down yet managed to stand up again. That is living proof of resilience. Each such memory is a building block for your self-belief and self-acceptance.

Guarding Against Cynicism

When going through repeated hardships, it is easy to become cynical. You might start believing the world is stacked against you or that there is no use in trying. However, cynicism tends to lock you into a state of hopelessness, making it harder to see possible solutions. Emotional resilience involves guarding against that mindset. You can admit the difficulties and still hold onto hope that you can adapt or find a new path. Hope is not blind optimism—it is the belief that with effort and time, change or recovery is possible.

Resilience in Relationships

Earlier in this book, we discussed how supportive relationships aid in self-acceptance. They also boost resilience. When you are part of a caring network, you do not face challenges alone. Friends or family can offer resources, suggestions, or simply a shoulder to cry on. But resilience is not one-sided; being supportive to others can also strengthen your own emotional health. Giving help often makes you realize you have skills or empathy you might have overlooked, reinforcing your sense of purpose and capability.

Avoiding Guilt Over Struggles

Many people feel guilty if they cannot "bounce back" quickly from sorrow or stress. They see others who appear to handle problems easily and think, "Why am I not as strong?" This comparison is unfair because everyone's journey is unique. Some hardships take a long time to heal. You might make progress, then suddenly feel like you are back at square one. That does not mean you are doing it wrong; it just means healing and growth do not always move in a straight line.

Tracking Progress

One way to appreciate your growing resilience is to track how you handle stress now compared to the past. Maybe a year ago, a small setback at work would ruin your whole week. Today, you feel upset for a day but then find a solution or accept it and move on. Or maybe you used to isolate yourself when sad, but now you reach out to a friend. These are signs of progress. When you notice these changes, you start to trust your ability to face challenges more confidently.

Maintaining Resilience Over the Long Term

Resilience is not a final destination. It is an ongoing practice. As you face bigger obstacles or life changes—like a career shift, parenthood, or aging—you will have to adapt your strategies. But each time you practice resilience, you make it a bit stronger. Think of it like a muscle that grows with use. The key is to keep using it, even when life is calm, so you stay prepared for the next wave of trouble.

Connecting Resilience to Self-Acceptance

Ultimately, emotional resilience and self-acceptance feed each other. When you accept yourself—flaws and all—you are less thrown by mistakes or harsh judgments from others. You do not see hardships as proof of being unworthy. Conversely, when you are resilient, you navigate those hardships without tearing down your self-esteem. You learn that tough moments are temporary dips, not permanent reflections of your identity.

This realization frees you to live more fully. You do not avoid challenges just because you fear failure or negative emotions. You try new things, have new experiences, and learn from what happens. The knowledge that you can bounce back keeps you from retreating into a shell of insecurity. Instead, you stand strong, arms open to the possibilities of life, willing to face whatever comes because you trust you have the inner tools to keep going.

Looking Ahead

Developing emotional resilience does not mean life will be free of problems. It means you can face them without losing yourself. As we continue this journey, the next chapters will bring more insights into how to maintain a growth mindset and balance caring for yourself with the responsibilities you carry. Each piece fits together—your self-belief, supportive relationships, resilience, and mindful living all play a part in creating a life where self-acceptance feels natural. Keep going, step by step, and remember that resilience grows each time you choose to get back up after falling.

CHAPTER 17: MAINTAINING A GROWTH MINDSET

A growth mindset is the belief that your skills, qualities, and intelligence can improve with effort. This idea suggests that you are not stuck at your current level; instead, you can keep learning and becoming better over time. It stands opposite to a fixed mindset, where a person might think abilities are unchangeable or that they are "born smart" or "bad at math" forever. When it comes to self-acceptance, a growth mindset helps you be kinder to yourself because you realize that mistakes and failures are not permanent labels—they are just steps on the path to growth.

In this chapter, we will look at what a growth mindset is, why it is important for self-acceptance, and how to maintain it over the long run.

What Is a Growth Mindset?

A growth mindset is a way of looking at challenges and opportunities with curiosity. You do not assume your abilities or intelligence are set in stone. Instead, you see them as areas you can develop. For instance, if you struggle with playing the piano, a fixed mindset might say, "I will never be a good piano player; I am just not musical." A growth mindset would say, "I can become better at piano if I practice and seek help when I need it."

Differences Between Growth and Fixed Mindsets

- **Response to Failure**: With a fixed mindset, failure feels like a dead end that defines who you are. With a growth mindset, failure is a sign that you need to adjust, try a new strategy, or practice more.
- **View of Effort**: People with a fixed mindset may see effort as a sign that they are not naturally good at something. People with a growth mindset understand that effort is part of improvement—if you invest time and energy, you can grow.
- **Attitude Toward Challenges**: A fixed mindset might lead you to avoid challenges to prevent embarrassment. A growth mindset makes you more willing to step into challenges, seeing them as chances to learn.

Why a Growth Mindset Supports Self-Acceptance

When you adopt a growth mindset, you become more patient with yourself. Instead of expecting instant perfection, you allow yourself space to be a learner. This perspective stops harsh self-criticism because you know that making mistakes is part of any journey. If you do poorly on a test or fail in a new project at work, you do not beat yourself up. You look for what you can do differently next time.

This shift in thinking aligns with self-acceptance because you begin to see that your worth is not tied to flawless performance. You are still worthy—even when you are in the messy middle of learning something new. By maintaining a growth mindset, you hold onto your sense of value, even during setbacks.

How a Growth Mindset Reduces Fear of Judgment

Fear of judgment often makes people shy away from new opportunities. If you believe failing a task would mean others see you as "not good enough," you might avoid trying altogether. But with a growth mindset, your focus is on the process rather than on others' opinions. You do your best, adjust, and keep going. This frees you from the worry of, "What will people think if I cannot do this perfectly?" because you know the real question is, "How can I improve and learn from this?"

Nurturing a Growth Mindset Daily

Embrace the Word "Yet"

One powerful way to encourage a growth mindset is to add the word "yet" when you talk about your current challenges. For example, if you find yourself saying, "I am not good at public speaking," change it to, "I am not good at public speaking yet." This simple word suggests that progress is possible. You might not be there today, but you are on your way.

Notice Fixed Mindset Thoughts

We all have moments when our thinking leans toward a fixed mindset. Maybe you think, "I will never understand math," or "I always fail at sports." When you catch these thoughts, pause and question them. Ask yourself, "Is that really true, or can I improve with practice and patience?" Over time, this awareness helps you break negative thought patterns.

Celebrate Small Progress

Growth is not just about big milestones. It also happens in small steps. Maybe you spoke up in a meeting even though you were anxious, or you learned a new chord on the guitar. Recognize these moments of progress. Saying "Good job for trying" or "I can see my progress" helps reinforce the belief that effort leads to improvement.

Seek Feedback

Feedback can be uncomfortable if you see it as criticism. But in a growth mindset, feedback is a gift—it shows you where you can get better. Whether from a teacher, a boss, or a friend, constructive feedback points out areas you might overlook on your own. That does not mean you have to accept all feedback blindly, but at least listen and see if there is something useful to learn.

Common Obstacles to a Growth Mindset

Perfectionism

Wanting to get everything right on the first try can harm a growth mindset. Perfectionism suggests that if you are not excellent immediately, you must be incompetent. But real growth rarely happens all at once. It is a gradual process, often with many missteps. Learning to see mistakes as natural can loosen perfectionism's hold.

Peer Pressure or Comparison

Sometimes, you might see a friend or coworker excel in a skill that you struggle with. It is easy to compare yourself and think, "They are just naturally better than I am." A growth mindset fights back by saying, "They might have practiced differently or have more experience. I can get there too, at my own pace." This way, you avoid using someone else's progress as proof of your own limitation.

Negative Self-Talk

Harsh thoughts about yourself can stifle growth. Telling yourself, "I am too old for this" or "I will never get better" can become a self-fulfilling prophecy. To maintain a growth mindset, be mindful of that negative inner voice and replace it with more balanced statements: "I may not learn as fast as I once did, but I can still improve if I keep trying."

Transforming Setbacks into Learning

When you face a setback, how you interpret it matters. A fixed mindset might label the experience as evidence that you are not talented or cut out for something. A growth mindset sees it as data—"This didn't go well, so what can I change next time?" This shift keeps your confidence from crumbling each time you encounter difficulty.

Reflect and Plan

After a setback, take a moment to reflect. Ask yourself what went wrong. Were you unprepared? Did you need different support or resources? Then plan your next step. Maybe you will ask for help from someone more experienced or study differently. This approach moves you forward instead of leaving you stuck in disappointment.

Accept Discomfort

Real growth often feels uncomfortable. You might worry about looking foolish or being judged. However, stepping out of your comfort zone is where learning happens. If something is too easy, you are likely not expanding your skills very much. Embrace the butterflies in your stomach as a sign you are stretching yourself.

The Role of Curiosity

A key ingredient of a growth mindset is curiosity. When you are curious, you look for new insights and experiences. You do not assume you have all the answers. Curiosity opens your mind to possibilities you might never explore otherwise. For instance, if you feel stuck in a career rut, a curious mindset might lead you to take a short course or shadow someone in a different department. You never know what you might discover if you keep an open mind.

Balancing a Growth Mindset with Self-Compassion

While it is good to push yourself, it is also important to be gentle when things do not happen as quickly as you hoped. Self-compassion reminds you that growth is a process, not a race. If you fail at a new skill, talk to yourself like you would a friend: "It is okay to stumble. You are learning. Keep going." This balance between a willingness to work hard and a kind inner voice keeps your morale high.

Bringing a Growth Mindset to Everyday Life

Learning in Ordinary Moments

Not every learning opportunity is big and formal. You might learn something new while cooking a meal, watching a documentary, or playing with a child. Maybe you figure out a faster way to do a chore, or you discover an unexpected interest just by being open to trying something different. By treating daily moments as small lessons, you keep your growth mindset active all the time.

Encouraging Others

When you see a friend or family member being hard on themselves, you can share the growth mindset perspective. Gently remind them that they can improve with effort and time. By supporting each other's growth, you create an environment where self-acceptance thrives—everyone feels free to try, fail, and learn without undue judgment.

Long-Term Goals

A growth mindset also shapes how you set goals. Instead of focusing only on big results—like "I must master the guitar in six months"—you aim for consistent progress: "I will practice guitar for 20 minutes a day and see where that takes me." This approach values the learning journey over a sudden leap to perfection. It also helps you adapt goals if needed, rather than quitting at the first sign of difficulty.

Handling Plateaus

Sometimes, your progress plateaus—you stop improving and feel stuck. This phase can be discouraging, and a fixed mindset might say, "I guess I have reached my limit." But in a growth mindset, you see a plateau as a sign to try a new method or seek fresh inspiration. Maybe you need a break, a different teacher, or a creative twist on practice. Plateaus are part of the learning curve, not proof that growth has ended.

How a Growth Mindset Affects Relationships

When you view yourself and others through a growth lens, you are more patient with mistakes or misunderstandings. You do not label people as "stubborn" or "clueless" without believing they can change. Instead, you recognize that humans are capable of learning and evolving in their thinking. This openness can lead to more forgiving and flexible relationships. If a friend makes a bad choice, you might say, "We can talk about it and grow through it together," rather than cutting them off entirely.

Dealing with Criticism from Others

It is one thing to handle your own negative thoughts; it is another to face criticism from people around you. Sometimes, others might doubt your ability to improve. They could say things like, "You will never change," or "Why bother?" Maintaining a growth mindset requires standing firm in your belief that change is possible. You might explain you are committed to learning, or you might simply keep doing the work and let your progress speak for itself.

Growth Mindset at Work or School

In a work or school environment, a growth mindset can help you see setbacks like a failed project or a poor grade as stepping stones. You view performance reviews or test results as feedback instead of final judgments on your ability. You also become more proactive in seeking resources, like tutors or mentors, to help you improve. Employers and teachers often appreciate individuals who display a willingness to grow rather than those who quit at the first obstacle.

Avoiding Burnout

While pushing yourself is key to growth, be mindful of burnout. Overloading your schedule with endless challenges might wear you down. A balanced growth mindset includes rest and reflection. Give yourself time to recharge, celebrate wins, and regroup before taking on the next challenge. Growth is a marathon, not a sprint.

Real-Life Stories

Think of people who overcame huge hurdles through consistent effort—like someone who learned to read as an adult, or an athlete who started out clumsy and became skilled through daily training. Their stories remind us that what seems impossible initially can become doable with steady work. Use these stories as motivation when your own challenges feel overwhelming.

Keeping Growth Going Over Time

A growth mindset is not a single choice you make once; it is a series of choices you make every day. You continually remind yourself that you can learn, adapt, and do better next time. When a door closes, you look for a window. When you hit a dead end, you turn around and find a different route. This mindset becomes a steady force in your life, pushing you to remain curious and unafraid of trying something new.

Conclusion: Your Ongoing Journey

Maintaining a growth mindset is a powerful tool in your journey of self-acceptance. It frees you from the prison of "I must be perfect right now" and replaces it with "I am growing all the time." That alone can reduce self-criticism and fear of failure. You become more flexible, curious, and willing to seek out opportunities for learning—even in areas where you once felt hopeless.

In our next chapter, we will explore balancing self-care with daily responsibilities, an important skill for preserving inner peace as you continue to grow. Just as a growth mindset helps you tackle challenges, knowing how to care for your emotional and physical well-being ensures you have enough energy and stability to keep moving forward. By combining these strengths, you create a supportive environment for ongoing self-acceptance and personal growth.

CHAPTER 18: BALANCING SELF-CARE AND RESPONSIBILITY

Life can be demanding. You may have responsibilities at work, at school, or at home—plus personal goals and relationships to maintain. It is easy to focus so heavily on meeting others' needs and fulfilling obligations that you forget to look after yourself. On the other hand, some people swing to the opposite extreme, tuning out responsibilities and focusing only on themselves. Balancing self-care with your duties is key to a healthy, satisfying life. It lets you meet your obligations without sacrificing your own well-being.

In this chapter, we will discuss why self-care is essential, how to create time for it despite a busy schedule, and how to handle guilt or stress that can arise when you feel pulled in multiple directions.

The Meaning of Self-Care

Self-care is any action you take to maintain or improve your mental, emotional, and physical health. It could be as simple as getting enough sleep, eating nutritious meals, or setting aside a few minutes to relax. It can also include hobbies that bring you joy, time with friends who recharge you, or even scheduling routine medical checkups.

Why Self-Care Matters

1. **Preventing Burnout**: If you keep giving energy to work, family, and other tasks without recharging, you risk burnout—feeling exhausted, unmotivated, and overwhelmed.
2. **Improving Mood**: Caring for yourself helps stabilize your emotions. When you are tired or stressed, you are more likely to feel irritable or sad. Self-care provides a balance that keeps your mood from dipping too low.
3. **Building Self-Respect**: Making room for your well-being signals to yourself that you matter. Over time, this message supports self-acceptance and confidence.

Common Myths About Self-Care

Some believe self-care is lazy or selfish. They might argue, "I do not have time for that," or "I should put others first." But self-care is not about ignoring responsibilities; it is about ensuring you have the energy and mental clarity to handle them well. Think of it like charging your phone—if you never charge it, it will die and be useless. Similarly, if you never recharge yourself, you will not be much help to anyone in the long run.

Identifying Your Responsibilities

Before you can balance self-care with responsibility, take stock of what you are responsible for in your life. This might include your job or schoolwork, household tasks, childcare, or caring for older family members. You might also have responsibilities to volunteer organizations or friends who rely on you for support. By listing these obligations, you see where your time and energy typically go.

Setting Priorities

Ask yourself which responsibilities are truly non-negotiable—like feeding your child or completing a major work project. Then see which ones might be flexible or shared with others. For instance, can you ask a roommate to help with cleaning, or can you delegate certain tasks at work? Identifying and sorting your responsibilities helps you find pockets of time or ways to reduce your load, making room for self-care.

Different Forms of Self-Care

Self-care is not just bubble baths and massages—though those can be nice if you enjoy them. People have different preferences and needs. Here are a few categories to consider):

- **Physical**: Exercise that suits your body, regular sleep patterns, nourishing meals.
- **Emotional**: Journaling, talking to a trusted friend, joining a support group, or practicing mindfulness.

- **Social**: Spending time with people who lift you up, or taking a break from social media if it stresses you.
- **Mental**: Reading, learning a new skill, engaging in puzzles or creative tasks that stimulate your mind.

Note that self-care should not feel like another chore. If you hate yoga, do not force yourself to do it just because others say it is relaxing. Choose activities that genuinely help you feel rested or fulfilled.

Creating a Self-Care Plan

Step 1: Assess Your Needs

Look at what areas of your life feel most strained. Are you physically exhausted, emotionally drained, or lacking social interaction? Understanding your specific needs guides you toward the right self-care activities.

Step 2: Pick Manageable Activities

Start small. If you rarely have time for yourself, consider taking a 10-minute walk each day or drinking a cup of tea in silence. Over time, you can expand to longer or more varied self-care activities. The key is consistency—regularly scheduling these moments so they become part of your routine.

Step 3: Set Boundaries

Self-care often requires saying no or reshaping your schedule. That might mean telling your boss you cannot work overtime every evening or telling a friend you cannot meet at the last minute if you already planned a night of rest. Boundaries ensure you protect the time you need to recharge.

Step 4: Track Your Feelings

Pay attention to how you feel after self-care. Do you notice less stress? Better sleep? A calmer mood? Tracking these changes, even in a simple journal entry, can motivate you to keep going when life gets busy.

Balancing Self-Care with Work or School

One challenge is that modern life often demands so much from us—emails, deadlines, exams—that self-care slides to the bottom of the priority list. But remember: ignoring your well-being can lead to burnout, which hurts your performance anyway. Balancing the two might look like:

- **Taking Micro-Breaks**: Stand up every hour to stretch or take a few deep breaths. Even a tiny pause can clear your head.
- **Planning Ahead**: If you know a big project is due next week, schedule times this week for both focused work and rest. By planning in advance, you avoid panic sprints where you drop all self-care to meet a deadline.
- **Discussing Flexibility**: If your workplace or school allows, see if you can adjust your schedule to fit in non-negotiable self-care. Maybe you arrive earlier so you can leave earlier for an exercise class, or you work from home one day a week to reduce commuting stress.

Handling Household and Family Responsibilities

For many, household chores or family care can consume a lot of time. If you share a home with family or roommates, consider dividing tasks fairly. Children can learn responsibility by doing age-appropriate chores. If a friend or relative always relies on you for favors, you might gently let them know you cannot always be available. Doing everything alone is a sure path to exhaustion.

It can also help to build small self-care habits around family time. For example, if you are cooking for your household, put on music you enjoy and treat it as a calming moment rather than a stressful task. If you have young children, maybe you set up a quiet coloring corner so they can do a calming activity while you read or stretch nearby.

Dealing with Guilt

Some people feel guilty when they carve out time for themselves, believing they are neglecting their duties or being selfish. Yet self-care is vital to keeping you capable of handling responsibilities in the long run. Remind yourself that you are allowed to need rest, and that taking a break is not the same as abandoning your tasks. It is about preserving your ability to do them well.

If guilt keeps rising, you can think: "By taking this 15 minutes to clear my head, I will be more patient with my children or more focused on my work." This shift in perspective can soothe the internal criticism that you are "slacking off."

Saying "No" When Necessary

Sometimes, the best self-care practice is simply learning to say "no." If your schedule is already full and someone requests a favor, you might have to decline. This does not make you a bad friend or coworker. It shows that you understand your limits and respect your need for balance. When you do say "yes," you can do so wholeheartedly, without resentment or burnout.

Self-Care During Difficult Times

When life hits hard—like a sudden illness, losing a job, or a relationship ending—self-care becomes even more crucial. Yet it is often the first thing people drop. You might think you have to handle the crisis non-stop. But even a few minutes of self-soothing, like a warm bath or a brief chat with a supportive friend, can keep you grounded. Trying to power through every moment of stress without breaks might worsen your mental or physical health, making it harder to overcome the crisis.

Overcoming Perfectionism in Self-Care

Ironically, some people approach self-care with perfectionism, feeling they must follow a perfect regimen of exercise, diet, and mindfulness. But that can add stress instead of removing it. Self-care should be about caring for yourself in ways that feel natural and comforting, not about meeting some rigid standard of "wellness." Be flexible. If one day you only have time for a quick 5-minute stretch or a single mindful breath, that is still better than nothing.

Supporting Self-Care in Relationships

If you have a partner or family, encourage them to practice self-care too. This helps prevent tension when one person gets burned out. You can coordinate schedules so each person gets some private relaxation time. You might also share certain self-care activities, like going for a walk together or cooking a healthy meal, so it doubles as bonding time.

Combining Self-Care with Personal Goals

Sometimes, we have personal goals like learning a new language, losing weight, or writing a book. These can feel like extra responsibilities, but if approached with a self-care mindset, they become fulfilling rather than draining. For example, if you want to learn a language, you can see it as an enjoyable break from daily stress—perhaps you watch cartoons or simple videos in that language for fun. If you want to exercise to get fit, pick activities you enjoy rather than forcing yourself through workouts you hate.

Creating Rituals or Routines

A helpful way to ensure self-care becomes part of your life is to create small rituals. For instance, you could start each morning with a moment of calm, where you sip your coffee slowly and note something you are grateful for. Or you end each evening with a short relaxation session—like gentle stretches or guided breathing. Over time, these rituals become second nature, giving you daily pockets of rest and reflection.

Checking In with Yourself

It is easy to get swept up in tasks and forget how you actually feel. Make a habit of checking in with yourself at least once a day. Close your eyes, take a slow breath, and ask: "How am I feeling right now—physically, mentally, emotionally?" If you notice tension or sadness, think about what self-care step might help. Even identifying the feeling can be a step toward easing it.

Handling Criticism

Sometimes, others will not understand your self-care decisions. They may question why you left a party early or turned down a request for help. They might say you are being too sensitive or that you should "just push through." Remember that you know your limits best. Politely but firmly explain that you are taking care of your well-being, or offer to help in a different way if possible. Not everyone will agree, but you do not need everyone's approval to protect your health.

Making Self-Care a Lifelong Habit

Balancing self-care and responsibility is not a one-time fix. Your needs and obligations will change as life changes—maybe you start a new job, move to a different city, or have children. In each new phase, you need to reassess how you can fit in self-care. Keep an open mind and adapt as you go along. Some seasons of life will allow more time for rest; others will be busier. The key is not to abandon self-care entirely, but to adjust its form to the situation.

Small Steps, Big Impact

If you are feeling overwhelmed by the idea of adding self-care on top of everything else, start with very small steps:

- Drink a full glass of water when you wake up.
- Take a 1-minute stretch break every few hours.
- Jot down one thing you are thankful for each day.
- Go outside for a short walk, even if it is just around the block.

Over time, these small habits can help you feel more grounded. You might then feel ready to expand to bigger self-care routines, like taking a weekly class or planning a monthly meet-up with close friends.

Connecting Back to Self-Acceptance

When you make time for self-care, you show yourself that you deserve care and attention. This act of kindness toward yourself directly strengthens your self-acceptance. It counters any negative beliefs that you must earn love by exhausting yourself for others. Instead, you realize you are worthy of rest, fun, and nourishment simply because you exist.

By balancing self-care with responsibility, you also avoid extremes—such as taking on too much or ignoring your duties altogether. This balanced approach supports healthy self-respect. You see that you can meet your obligations while also treating yourself kindly. Over time, this balance can become second nature, making your life more joyful and less stressful.

Conclusion: Walking the Middle Path

Life often pulls us in many directions. Work, family, friends, and personal goals all demand our time. By weaving self-care into your daily routine, you ensure you do not lose yourself in the process. This balance is not always easy, and you may slip sometimes, either by neglecting your well-being or by dropping important tasks. But each slip is an opportunity to re-evaluate and find a steadier path forward.

In the next chapters, we will continue exploring tools to strengthen your sense of self and your ability to handle life's demands. We will look at celebrating small wins and, finally, how to carry all these lessons forward into a future of ongoing self-acceptance. For now, remind yourself that true balance can be found when you treat your duties seriously, but also honor your need for rest, play, and personal growth. By caring for yourself, you invest in a happier, healthier you—and that ultimately benefits everyone around you as well.

CHAPTER 19: CARRYING SELF-ACCEPTANCE FORWARD

Reaching the end of this book does not mean you have fully mastered self-acceptance. Instead, think of this as a checkpoint on a life-long journey. You have learned about understanding your worth, facing negative self-talk, embracing your flaws, building emotional resilience, and more. Now, the question is: how do you carry these lessons forward into your future, ensuring that you keep growing and remain at peace with who you are?

This final chapter will focus on integrating all the tools we have explored and turning them into daily habits that can guide you through both routine days and challenging times. We will also talk about how to adjust your mindset as life changes, because self-acceptance is not a one-size-fits-all solution. It evolves as you evolve.

Reflecting on the Journey

Before moving forward, it helps to reflect on how far you have come. Even reading through these chapters is a form of action—you have invested time and energy in understanding yourself better. Maybe you have noticed changes, like being kinder to yourself after a mistake or speaking up more confidently in certain situations. Or perhaps you are just starting to see small shifts in how you think about your worth.

Take a moment to appreciate that reflection. It is similar to the idea of celebrating small wins from the previous chapter. Recognizing the distance you have already traveled builds faith that you can continue onward.

Designing Your Personal Plan

Reviewing Key Lessons

We have covered many topics: self-compassion, boundaries, letting go of perfectionism, healing past hurt, building supportive relationships, developing a growth mindset, practicing mindfulness, managing stress, and more. It might help to list out the strategies or ideas that resonated most with you. Which chapters spoke to your current needs? Which exercises seemed most helpful?

By highlighting your favorite tools, you create a personal "menu" of strategies you can reach for when life challenges you. You do not have to remember every detail of every chapter. It is enough to recall that, for example, mindfulness calms your racing thoughts, or setting boundaries keeps you from feeling overwhelmed, or celebrating small wins boosts your motivation.

Making Time for Practice

Self-acceptance does not maintain itself automatically. You need to practice the skills that keep you grounded. This might involve scheduling a few minutes each day or each week to check in with yourself. You could review your boundaries, write in a journal about your recent wins and challenges, or do a mindfulness exercise. By setting aside even a little time, you keep these lessons fresh, preventing old habits from creeping back unnoticed.

Adapting to Life Changes

Life is full of transitions—maybe you switch jobs, move to a new place, start a new relationship, or face a loss. Each transition can test your self-acceptance in different ways. For instance, when you move to a new city, you might feel lonely or uncertain about making friends. Remember to revisit the chapters about supportive relationships or about facing fear and self-doubt. Or if you step into a leadership role at work, you can recall the lessons on building confidence and handling stress. Adapting means you continuously reshape your self-acceptance practices to suit new circumstances.

Keeping a Forward-Looking Mindset

While reflecting on the past is helpful, dwelling too much on mistakes or regrets can stall you. Self-acceptance includes accepting that your past self did the best it could with what it knew at the time. Now, you can look forward, focusing on what you can do today and tomorrow. This forward-looking mindset is anchored in the idea that you are always learning and evolving. You are not defined by who you were last year or last week. You can continue to grow into the person you want to be.

Supporting Yourself Through Setbacks

No matter how much you practice self-acceptance, you will still face setbacks. You might find yourself returning to old habits of negative self-talk or feeling unworthy after a big disappointment. This is normal. The key is to recognize the setback, remind yourself it does not undo your progress, and use your tools to bounce back. For instance, if you catch your inner critic telling you, "You failed again; you are hopeless," you can counter with self-compassion: "I had a tough day, but this does not define me. I can learn and try again." Over time, these setbacks become temporary bumps rather than deep pits you cannot climb out of.

Building a Support Network

Throughout this book, we have seen how supportive relationships can reinforce your self-acceptance. As you move forward, keep nurturing the connections that help you grow. Surround yourself with people who respect your boundaries, celebrate your small wins, and believe in your ability to learn. If you do not have such people in your life right now, consider looking for communities—online or in person—focused on personal growth or shared interests. A supportive network can serve as a safety net when you falter and a cheer squad when you thrive.

Passing the Torch

As you deepen your self-acceptance, you might notice changes in how you interact with others. You could become more patient, more understanding, and more encouraging. This ripple effect can inspire friends or family to embark on their own journeys of self-growth. While you are not responsible for anyone else's path, being open about your process and offering gentle advice can help them see that self-acceptance is possible.

At the same time, remember to respect their choices. Not everyone is ready to work on self-acceptance at the same pace. Offer your experience if they show interest, but do not push them or criticize if they are not on the same page. Your example alone can be a powerful spark of hope.

Continuing Education

Self-acceptance is a vast topic, and this book is just one resource. If you want to keep learning, you can explore other materials—like podcasts on mental health, articles about personal growth, or courses on emotional intelligence. You might also consider therapy or coaching if you want more personalized guidance. The idea is to keep feeding your mind with wisdom that supports your journey, rather than letting it fade when you close this book.

Embracing Impermanence

A big part of self-acceptance is embracing the fact that everything changes. Your feelings, your body, your relationships—they all evolve over time. Instead of fighting that reality, you can flow with it. This means letting yourself be flexible, adjusting your goals when you need to, and allowing people around you to change without clinging to an older version of them. Impermanence is not something to fear; it is part of the beauty of growth. It means you are never stuck in a single state.

Checking In with Your Inner Voice

By now, you have spent time working on quieting negative self-talk or turning it into more supportive inner dialogue. Keep an ear out for that voice going forward. If you hear it slip into harsh judgments—like labeling yourself "stupid" for an honest mistake—pause and correct it gently. Say, "I made a mistake. That is normal. Let's figure out a way to fix it." Over time, this supportive voice becomes more natural, but it requires ongoing attention to keep it from reverting to negativity.

Making Peace with Imperfection

One theme that has come up repeatedly is that no one is perfect. Perfectionism can block self-acceptance by insisting you must never slip up. As you move forward, it helps to keep reminding yourself that a little messiness is part of being human. Maybe you forget an appointment or lose your temper occasionally—that does not erase your worth. If you notice perfectionistic thoughts creeping back, recall the chapters about releasing the need to be flawless. Accepting imperfection frees you to learn and adapt, rather than punishing yourself for every minor error.

Celebrating Ongoing Victories

We talked about celebrating small wins. This habit should continue beyond the period of reading this book. Each time you move past a challenge—like having a tough conversation, finishing a difficult task, or showing compassion to someone who hurt you—take a moment to acknowledge it. This is how you keep your energy and optimism alive.

If possible, share these victories with friends or a journal. A simple remark like, "I finally asked for help at work today; it felt scary, but I did it!" can reinforce the significance of that step. Over months and years, these repeated acknowledgments form a narrative of someone who keeps growing and learning, which supports your self-acceptance at a deep level.

Adjusting to Setbacks in Motivation

Even the most dedicated people go through slumps. You might feel an ebb in motivation, as if you are tired of focusing on personal growth. That is normal. Sometimes you need a period of rest from conscious self-work, allowing your mind to breathe. During those times, keep a gentle baseline—maybe you still do a quick daily check-in or practice small self-care activities. Once you feel re-energized, you can return to deeper exploration. Self-acceptance does not mean you have to be in constant self-improvement mode. It is about honoring the rhythm of your life.

Setting an Example for Younger Generations

If you have children, nieces, nephews, or younger siblings, remember that they often learn self-acceptance (or self-criticism) by watching adults. When they see you treat yourself kindly after a mistake, they pick up on that. When they see you set healthy boundaries or take time for self-care, they learn that they too can prioritize their well-being. Modeling these behaviors is a powerful way to influence the next generation, possibly sparing them from some struggles with low self-esteem.

Looking Back and Looking Ahead

It can be helpful to mark each year or season with a short reflection. You might ask, "How have I grown in self-acceptance in the past year? What challenges arose, and how did I handle them differently than before?" Then you can look ahead: "What areas of my life need more nurturing? Where can I apply these tools more effectively?" This annual or seasonal check-in keeps your journey active rather than something you read about once and then forgot.

Embracing the Ongoing Nature of Growth

Some people get frustrated that self-acceptance is not a "one and done" achievement. They might say, "I worked on this, why is it not fixed yet?" But acceptance is not about fixing; it is about understanding and being at peace with who you are, day by day, even as you improve. It is like maintaining a garden—it requires weeding, watering, and care across seasons. The garden never stays exactly the same, and that is okay. It will bloom anew in different forms, reflecting the changes in weather and soil.

Conclusion: A Life of Self-Acceptance

We have reached the final chapter of this book, but your own story continues. Self-acceptance is the thread that weaves through all your experiences. You now have a collection of tools—mindfulness, self-compassion, boundary setting, resilience, growth mindset, celebrating small wins, and more. By using these tools, you can face challenges without losing your sense of worth, adapt to life's changes with more grace, and find peace in who you are each day.

Remember that none of this requires you to be perfect. The person you are right now is worthy of kindness and understanding, just as you were when you started reading. The main difference is that you have more awareness and skills to navigate the ups and downs of life. Each time you apply what you learned, you strengthen the bond you have with yourself.

As you move forward, keep these core ideas in mind:

1. **Self-acceptance is a journey**—it grows as you do.
2. **Mistakes and setbacks** are part of learning, not signs of failure.

3. **Healthy boundaries** and supportive relationships help you stay true to yourself.
4. **Taking care of your mental and emotional well-being** is a responsibility, not a luxury.
5. **Celebrating small wins** keeps you motivated along the way.

There will be moments when self-doubt returns. There will be days you slip into old habits of negative thinking or pushing yourself too hard. That is part of being human. But now you have the knowledge to recognize those pitfalls and the power to choose differently. You can remind yourself: "I am allowed to be a work in progress. I accept myself for who I am, while still striving to grow."

I hope the insights and practices in these chapters help you find lasting peace and confidence. As you continue your life, remember to pause once in a while to see how far you have come. Even small steps, taken regularly, can lead to big transformations. May your journey of self-acceptance guide you to a life filled with understanding, compassion—both for yourself and for others—and the unwavering sense that you are worthy of love and respect, today and every day forward.

Printed in Great Britain
by Amazon